CLINICAL RED FLAGS, PEARLS, AND PITFALLS

A Comprehensive Guide for Medical Students and Clinicians

Dr Essam Abdelhakim

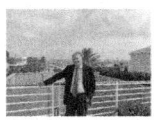

CONTENTS

INTRODUCTION

*"**Essential Clinical Scenarios and Red Flags**" is designed to provide a comprehensive yet practical guide for medical students, general practitioners (GPs), international medical graduates (IMGs), residents, and emergency physicians.*

The core of this book lies in **case-based learning**—an approach that mirrors real-world medical practice.

Each chapter is structured around carefully crafted clinical scenarios that represent common, complex, and critical presentations across a broad spectrum of specialties.

These scenarios not only provide an in-depth understanding of the conditions presented, but also highlight **red flags**—key warning signs that indicate when a condition may be urgent, severe, or life-threatening.

Recognizing these red flags early can significantly impact diagnosis, management, and patient outcomes, especially in emergency situations or in the context of urgent care.

NEUROLOGICAL RED FLAGS 1

- 1. Sudden, Severe Headache ("Thunderclap Headache")

Case 1: The Headache that Struck Like Lightning

Scenario: *A 40-year-old woman presents to the emergency department with a sudden onset severe headache that began during exercise.*

She describes it as "the worst headache of my life." She is photophobic and mildly nauseated, but her neurological exam is unremarkable.

- **Red Flag**: Thunderclap headache
- **Differential Diagnosis**:
    - Subarachnoid hemorrhage (SAH)
    - Cerebral venous sinus thrombosis
    - Pituitary apoplexy
    - Cervical artery dissection
- **Next Steps**:
    - Immediate non-contrast CT brain
    - If CT is negative and suspicion remains high → lumbar puncture to look for xanthochromia
- **Pearl**: A normal neurological exam does **not** rule out SAH
- **Pitfall**: Attributing symptoms to migraine without proper evaluation

- 2. New-Onset Seizure

Case 2: First-Time Fit in a Young Adult

Scenario: *A 25-year-old man collapses in a store with limb jerking lasting 2 minutes, followed by confusion.*
No history of epilepsy. He had a recent headache and mild fever.

- **Red Flag**: New-onset seizure in an adult
- **Differential Diagnosis**:
    - Structural lesion (e.g. tumor, stroke)
    - CNS infection (e.g. encephalitis)
    - Metabolic derangements (e.g. hyponatremia, hypoglycemia)
    - Substance withdrawal/toxicity
- **Next Steps**:
    - CT or MRI brain
    - Blood tests (including glucose, electrolytes, toxicology)
    - Lumbar puncture if infection is suspected
    - EEG
- **Pearl**: First-time seizures warrant urgent imaging and full workup
- **Pitfall**: Dismissing it as "just stress" or sleep deprivation

- 3. Acute Focal Neurological Deficit

Case 3: The Sudden Weakness

Scenario: *A 67-year-old man presents with sudden onset left arm and leg weakness, slurred speech, and facial droop. Symptoms started 1* *hour ago.*

He has a history of hypertension and atrial fibrillation.

- **Red Flag**: Acute unilateral weakness
- **Differential Diagnosis**:
    - Ischemic stroke
    - Hemorrhagic stroke
    - Seizure with Todd's paresis
    - Hypoglycemia
- **Next Steps**:
    - Immediate **CT brain** to rule out hemorrhage
    - If ischemic stroke suspected and within 4.5 hours → consider **thrombolysis**
    - Blood glucose check (to exclude hypoglycemia mimic)
- **Pearl**: "Time is brain"—stroke protocols must be initiated fast
- **Pitfall**: Waiting too long for imaging or underestimating subtle symptoms

- 4. Altered Mental Status

Case 4: Grandma Isn't Herself Today

Scenario: *An 80-year-old woman with a known history of diabetes is brought by family due to confusion for 1 day.*

She is lethargic, disoriented, and has mild dehydration. No focal neurological deficit.

- **Red Flag**: Sudden confusion in an elderly patient
- **Differential Diagnosis**:
    - Hypoglycemia or hyperosmolar hyperglycemic state (HHS)

- Sepsis (e.g. UTI, pneumonia)
- Stroke (esp. posterior circulation)
- Medication toxicity (e.g. benzodiazepines)

- **Next Steps**:
  - Blood glucose, electrolytes, urinalysis, CXR
  - CT brain if focal signs, trauma, or persistent AMS
- **Pearl**: Always think metabolic or infectious in elderly with acute confusion
- **Pitfall**: Mislabeling as dementia without investigating reversible causes

- 5. Sudden Monocular Vision Loss

Case 5: The Black Curtain

Scenario: *A 59-year-old man complains of sudden painless loss of vision in his right eye.*

He describes it like "a curtain came down." He is hypertensive and has a history of smoking.

- **Red Flag**: Sudden painless monocular vision loss
- **Differential Diagnosis**:
  - Central retinal artery occlusion (CRAO)
  - Amaurosis fugax
  - Retinal detachment
  - Optic neuritis
- **Next Steps**:
  - Urgent fundoscopy: cherry red spot suggests CRAO
  - Immediate referral to ophthalmology/stroke team

- ◦ Work-up for carotid stenosis, cardiac emboli
- **Pearl**: CRAO is a form of stroke—treat urgently
- **Pitfall**: Misdiagnosed as ocular migraine or dry eye

- 6. Neck Stiffness With Fever Or Photophobia

Case 6: A Headache with a Warning

Scenario: *A 22-year-old university student presents with headache, fever, photophobia, and vomiting.*
He has a stiff neck and a purpuric rash on his legs.

- **Red Flag**: Headache + fever + neck stiffness
- **Differential Diagnosis**:
  - ◦ Bacterial meningitis (e.g. Neisseria meningitidis)
  - ◦ Viral meningitis
  - ◦ Encephalitis
  - ◦ Subarachnoid hemorrhage (if no fever)
- **Next Steps**:
  - ◦ Immediate **empiric IV antibiotics**
  - ◦ CT brain if altered mental status before LP
  - ◦ Lumbar puncture when safe
- **Pearl**: In meningitis, treat first—don't delay antibiotics for LP
- **Pitfall**: Waiting for labs or LP before starting treatment

- 7. Back Pain With Bladder/Bowel Dysfunction

Case 7: The Back Pain That Couldn't Wait

Scenario: *A 52-year-old man presents with severe lower back pain for 3 days, now with difficulty urinating and numbness in the perineal region.*

He also complains of weakness in both legs.

- **Red Flag**: Back pain + urinary retention + saddle anesthesia
- **Diagnosis: Cauda equina syndrome**
- **Next Steps**:
    - Urgent **MRI spine**
    - Immediate referral to neurosurgery or spinal surgery
    - Catheterize for retention
- **Pearl**: Ask about **saddle anesthesia** in any severe back pain case
- **Pitfall**: Misdiagnosing as simple sciatica or disc herniation without red flag screening

CARDIOLOGY RED FLAGS

- 1. Chest Pain Suggestive Of Acute Coronary Syndrome (Acs)

Case 1: Crushing Chest Pain

Scenario: *A 60-year-old man presents with central chest pain radiating to his left arm, associated with sweating and nausea.*

He has a history of hypertension and type 2 diabetes.

- **Red Flag**: Chest pain with radiation + diaphoresis
- **Differential Diagnosis**:
    - Acute coronary syndrome (STEMI/NSTEMI)
    - Aortic dissection
    - Pulmonary embolism
    - Pericarditis
- **Next Steps**:
    - ECG within 10 minutes
    - Cardiac troponins
    - Aspirin, oxygen, nitrates, morphine as appropriate
    - Cardiology referral ± PCI if STEMI
- **Pearl**: "Time is myocardium"—never delay ECG in chest pain
- **Pitfall**: Atypical presentations in elderly or diabetics may lack classic pain

- 2. Sudden Onset Of Severe Tearing Chest/Back Pain

Case 2: The Chest Pain that Ripped Apart

Scenario: *A 72-year-old man with hypertension presents with sudden severe tearing chest pain radiating to the back.*

He is pale and has unequal blood pressures in his arms.

- **Red Flag**: Tearing chest pain + unequal limb BPs
- **Diagnosis: Aortic dissection**
- **Differential Diagnosis**:
  - Myocardial infarction
  - Pulmonary embolism
  - Esophageal rupture
- **Next Steps**:
  - Urgent CT angiography of the aorta
  - IV beta-blockers to reduce BP/HR
  - Cardiothoracic surgery consult
- **Pearl**: Dissections can mimic MI—don't thrombolyse without confirming
- **Pitfall**: Missing BP discrepancy or sudden back pain

- 3. Syncope With Exertion Or Palpitations

Case 3: Fainting on the Field

Scenario: *A 17-year-old football player collapses during practice. He had brief palpitations before fainting.*

No seizure-like activity. He regains consciousness quickly.

- **Red Flag**: Syncope with exertion + palpitations
- **Differential Diagnosis**:
  - Hypertrophic cardiomyopathy (HCM)

9

- Arrhythmogenic right ventricular cardiomyopathy
- Long QT syndrome or other channelopathies
- Ventricular tachyarrhythmia
- **Next Steps:**
  - ECG + echocardiogram
  - Consider 24-hour Holter or stress testing
  - Refer to cardiology/genetic counselling if hereditary disease suspected
- **Pearl:** Syncope during exertion is cardiac until proven otherwise
- **Pitfall:** Labeling it as vasovagal without full cardiac workup

- 4. Shortness Of Breath + Orthopnea + Bilateral Leg Swelling

Case 4: The Breathless Man

Scenario: *A 68-year-old man presents with progressive shortness of breath, especially at night.*

He sleeps propped up on 3 pillows. On exam, there are bilateral basal crackles and pedal edema.

- **Red Flag**: Orthopnea + peripheral edema + fatigue
- **Diagnosis: Heart failure (likely HFrEF)**
- **Differential Diagnosis**:
  - COPD/asthma
  - Pulmonary hypertension
  - Renal failure
- **Next Steps**:
  - BNP/NT-proBNP
  - ECG + echocardiogram
  - CXR (cardiomegaly, pulmonary edema)
  - Diuretics and ACE inhibitors
- **Pearl**: Orthopnea and PND are classic for left-sided heart failure
- **Pitfall**: Assuming it's just COPD in older smokers

- 5. Palpitations With Hemodynamic Instability

Case 5: The Racing Heart

Scenario: *A 45-year-old woman with a history of anxiety presents with palpitations and dizziness.*

On exam: HR 180, BP 85/60, ECG shows narrow complex tachycardia.

- **Red Flag**: Palpitations + hypotension + altered consciousness
- **Diagnosis: SVT with hemodynamic instability**
- **Differential Diagnosis**:
  - AVNRT, AVRT
  - Atrial fibrillation with RVR
  - Ventricular tachycardia (if wide QRS)
- **Next Steps**:
  - Immediate synchronized cardioversion if unstable
  - If stable: vagal maneuvers → adenosine → rate control
  - Further workup for triggers (thyroid, caffeine, etc.)
- **Pearl**: Any tachycardia with hypotension = emergency
- **Pitfall**: Waiting too long to cardiovert in unstable patient

- 6. Chest Pain With Recent Immobilization Or Surgery

Case 6: The Silent Clot

Scenario: *A 35-year-old woman, 2 weeks post-C-section, presents with sudden pleuritic chest pain, shortness of breath, and tachycardia. She is mildly hypoxic on room air.*

- **Red Flag**: Sudden pleuritic pain + hypoxia + recent surgery
- **Diagnosis: Pulmonary embolism**
- **Differential Diagnosis**:
  - Pneumonia
  - MI
  - Pneumothorax
- **Next Steps**:
  - Wells score/D-dimer → CTPA
  - Start anticoagulation if high suspicion
  - Monitor oxygen saturation and hemodynamics
- **Pearl**: Always think PE in sudden dyspnea + risk factor (e.g. surgery, OCPs)
- **Pitfall**: Attributing it to post-op pain or anxiety

- 7. Bradycardia With Syncope Or Confusion

Case 7: The Slow Heart

Scenario: *A 75-year-old man with known ischemic heart disease presents with confusion and near-syncope.*

His pulse is 35 bpm. ECG shows complete heart block.

- **Red Flag**: Bradycardia + dizziness/syncope
- **Diagnosis: Complete (third-degree) AV block**
- **Differential Diagnosis**:
    - Sick sinus syndrome
    - Medication toxicity (e.g. beta-blockers)
    - Acute inferior MI
- **Next Steps**:
    - Stop AV-nodal blocking drugs
    - Temporary pacing if unstable
    - Permanent pacemaker referral
- **Pearl**: Slow heart + symptoms = pacemaker unless reversible cause
- **Pitfall**: Assuming it's benign aging or dehydration

- 8. Sudden Cardiac Arrest In Young Athlete Or Postpartum Woman

Case 8: Collapse in a Crowd

Scenario: *A 28-year-old postpartum woman suddenly collapses while walking in a shopping mall. Bystanders initiate CPR.*

On arrival, rhythm is pulseless VT.

- **Red Flag**: Sudden cardiac arrest in a young person
- **Differential Diagnosis**:
    - Cardiomyopathy (e.g. postpartum)
    - Channelopathies (e.g. long QT, Brugada)
    - Massive PE
    - Coronary anomaly
- **Next Steps**:
    - ACLS + defibrillation
    - Cardiac workup: echo, coronary angiography, MRI
    - Genetic testing/counseling if inherited arrhythmia suspected
- **Pearl**: Consider genetic and structural causes in young SCA survivors
- **Pitfall**: Focusing only on coronary artery disease

RESPIRATORY RED FLAGS

- 1. Sudden Onset Dyspnea With Chest Pain

Case 1: The Post-Flight Emergency

Scenario: *A 32-year-old woman develops sudden shortness of breath and pleuritic chest pain two days after returning from a long-haul flight.*

She is mildly tachycardic and has an SpO$_2$ of 90% on room air.

- **Red Flag**: Sudden dyspnea + pleuritic pain + recent immobilization (flight)
- **Differential Diagnosis**:
    - **Pulmonary embolism**
    - Pneumothorax
    - Pneumonia
    - MI
- **Next Steps**:
    - Calculate Wells Score
    - D-dimer if low-to-intermediate risk
    - CTPA if high risk or positive D-dimer
    - Start anticoagulation if PE suspected
- **Pearl**: Always suspect PE in sudden dyspnea + risk factor (immobilization, surgery, pregnancy, OCP)
- **Pitfall**: Dismissing symptoms as anxiety or "jet lag"

- 2. Hemoptysis With Weight Loss

Case 2: The Coughing Smoker

Scenario: *A 58-year-old man with a 40-pack-year smoking history presents with hemoptysis, chronic cough, and recent unintentional weight loss.*

He looks cachectic and has digital clubbing.

- **Red Flag**: Hemoptysis + weight loss + smoking history
- **Differential Diagnosis**:
  - **Lung cancer**
  - Tuberculosis
  - Bronchiectasis
  - Fungal infection
- **Next Steps**:
  - Chest X-ray → CT chest
  - Sputum cytology & AFB
  - Refer to pulmonology/oncology
- **Pearl**: Hemoptysis in an older smoker = cancer until proven otherwise
- **Pitfall**: Treating empirically for bronchitis without further evaluation

- 3. Stridor And Drooling In Febrile Child

Case 3: The Drooling Toddler

Scenario: *A 3-year-old child is brought to the ED with high fever, drooling, muffled voice, and sitting in a tripod position.*

Stridor is heard on inspiration.

- **Red Flag**: Acute stridor + drooling + tripod posture
- **Differential Diagnosis**:
  - **Epiglottitis**
  - Croup
  - Foreign body

- ◦ Bacterial tracheitis
- **Next Steps**:
  - ◦ Do **not** examine throat
  - ◦ Keep child calm
  - ◦ Call anaesthetics + ENT for controlled airway management
  - ◦ IV antibiotics (e.g. ceftriaxone)
- **Pearl**: Drooling and tripod posture = airway emergency
- **Pitfall**: Forcing child to lie down or examining throat can provoke arrest

- 4. Rapidly Increasing Breathlessness + Pink Frothy Sputum

Case 4: The Overloaded Heart

Scenario: *A 72-year-old man with a history of MI and heart failure presents with acute dyspnea and pink frothy sputum.*

He is hypoxic and tachypneic with bilateral crackles on auscultation.

- **Red Flag**: Acute pulmonary edema signs (frothy sputum + hypoxia + orthopnea)
- **Differential Diagnosis**:
  - **Acute decompensated heart failure**
  - Pulmonary embolism
  - ARDS
  - Pneumonia
- **Next Steps**:
  - High-flow oxygen or CPAP
  - IV diuretics (furosemide)
  - Nitrates ± morphine
  - Monitor closely in HDU/ICU setting
- **Pearl**: Orthopnea and frothy sputum = classic signs of acute pulmonary edema
- **Pitfall**: Missing cardiac cause in a respiratory presentation

- 5. Fever + Night Sweats + Cough + Travel History

Case 5: The Persistent Cough

Scenario: *A 29-year-old medical student recently returned from India. He presents with a persistent cough, low-grade fever, and night sweats.*

His chest X-ray shows upper lobe infiltrates and cavitations.

- **Red Flag**: Fever + night sweats + cough + upper lobe infiltrates
- **Differential Diagnosis**:
  - **Tuberculosis**
  - Lung abscess
  - Sarcoidosis
  - Fungal infection (e.g. histoplasmosis)
- **Next Steps**:
  - Isolate the patient
  - Sputum for AFB x3
  - TB PCR/NAAT
  - Notify public health
- **Pearl**: Always ask travel and exposure history in respiratory complaints
- **Pitfall**: Delayed isolation leads to nosocomial transmission

- 6. Sudden Onset Dyspnea + Hyperresonance

Case 6: The Collapsed Lung

Scenario: *A tall, thin 19-year-old male presents with sudden onset of left-sided pleuritic chest pain and shortness of breath.*

On exam: trachea deviated to the right, hyperresonant left hemithorax, absent breath sounds.

- **Red Flag**: Sudden dyspnea + hyperresonance + tracheal deviation
- **Diagnosis**: **Tension pneumothorax**
- **Differential Diagnosis**:
  - Simple pneumothorax
  - PE
  - Acute asthma attack
- **Next Steps**:
  - Immediate needle decompression (2nd ICS midclavicular)
  - Followed by chest tube insertion
- **Pearl**: Tension pneumothorax is a **clinical** diagnosis— don't wait for imaging
- **Pitfall**: Delaying intervention while waiting for CXR

- 7. Rapid Respiratory Deterioration + Ground-Glass Opacities

Case 7: The Breathless Pandemic Patient

Scenario: *A 55-year-old man with COVID-19 presents with increasing oxygen requirement, worsening dyspnea, and bilateral ground-glass infiltrates on CT chest.*

SpO_2 86% on 15L non-rebreather.

- **Red Flag**: Hypoxia not responding to high-flow O_2 + bilateral infiltrates
- **Differential Diagnosis**:
  - **ARDS (Acute Respiratory Distress Syndrome)**
  - Severe COVID-19 pneumonia
  - Pneumocystis jirovecii pneumonia (if immunocompromised)
  - Influenza A pneumonia
- **Next Steps**:
  - Admit to ICU for advanced respiratory support
  - Consider proning and mechanical ventilation
  - Dexamethasone, anticoagulation, and supportive care
- **Pearl**: Silent hypoxia in COVID-19 patients can precede rapid deterioration
- **Pitfall**: Delaying escalation to ICU or underestimating oxygen demand

- 8. Chronic Productive Cough + Clubbing + Recurrent Infections

Case 8: The Wet Cough

Scenario: *A 30-year-old woman presents with chronic productive cough, digital clubbing, and multiple previous admissions for chest infections since childhood.*

- **Red Flag**: Chronic wet cough + clubbing + recurrent infections
- **Diagnosis: Bronchiectasis**
- **Differential Diagnosis**:
  - Cystic fibrosis
  - COPD
  - Chronic aspiration
  - Primary ciliary dyskinesia
- **Next Steps**:
  - High-resolution CT chest
  - Sputum culture
  - Physiotherapy referral
  - Consider long-term antibiotics
- **Pearl**: Chronic cough + clubbing = investigate for structural lung disease
- **Pitfall**: Labeling it as simple asthma or smoker's cough without imaging

GASTROINTESTINAL RED FLAGS

- 1. Hematemesis Or Coffee Ground Vomiting

Case 1: The Bleeding Ulcer

Scenario: *A 64-year-old man with a history of NSAID use presents with vomiting of dark blood (coffee ground material) and lightheadedness.*

He is tachycardic and his BP is 95/60 mmHg.

- **Red Flag**: Hematemesis + hypotension
- **Differential Diagnosis**:
  - **Peptic ulcer bleeding**
  - Esophageal varices
  - Gastric cancer
  - Mallory-Weiss tear
- **Next Steps**:
  - ABC approach
  - IV fluids, crossmatch blood
  - Urgent upper GI endoscopy
  - Start IV PPI (e.g., omeprazole)
- **Pearl**: Coffee ground vomitus suggests **upper GI bleeding**, possibly slower or partial digestion of blood
- **Pitfall**: Underestimating bleeding severity in elderly or patients on beta-blockers

- 2. Progressive Dysphagia

Case 2: The Swallowing Struggle

Scenario: *A 58-year-old man reports progressive difficulty swallowing solids, then liquids, over several months.*

He has lost 8 kg unintentionally and often regurgitates undigested food.

- **Red Flag**: Dysphagia + weight loss + progression from solids to liquids
- **Differential Diagnosis**:
  - **Esophageal carcinoma**
  - Achalasia
  - Peptic stricture
  - Esophagitis
- **Next Steps**:
  - Urgent upper GI endoscopy
  - Barium swallow
  - CT scan of chest and abdomen (staging if cancer)
- **Pearl**: Progressive dysphagia = **malignancy until proven otherwise**
- **Pitfall**: Assuming it's GERD and prescribing PPIs without investigating

- 3. Painless Jaundice

Case 3: The Yellow Businessman

Scenario: *A 65-year-old man presents with yellowing of the skin and eyes, dark urine, pale stools, and no abdominal pain. He has lost 6 kg over 2 months.*

On exam, he has a palpable gallbladder.

- **Red Flag**: Painless jaundice + weight loss + palpable gallbladder (Courvoisier's sign)
- **Differential Diagnosis**:

- **Pancreatic head cancer**
- Cholangiocarcinoma
- Stricture from chronic pancreatitis

- **Next Steps**:
  - LFTs (obstructive pattern)
  - Ultrasound liver + biliary tree
  - CT pancreas ± MRCP
  - Refer to GI oncology

- **Pearl**: Painless jaundice is a hallmark of **pancreatic or biliary malignancy**

- **Pitfall**: Dismissing jaundice as "hepatitis" without full workup

- 4. Iron-Deficiency Anemia In Men Or Postmenopausal Women

Case 4: The Fatigued Accountant

Scenario: *A 50-year-old man is found to have Hb 9 g/dL, MCV 72, and ferritin 5. He denies any overt bleeding.*

Occult blood test is positive. No NSAID use.

- **Red Flag**: Unexplained iron-deficiency anemia
- **Differential Diagnosis**:
  - **Colorectal cancer**
  - Angiodysplasia
  - Hookworm (if endemic)
  - Peptic ulcer
- **Next Steps**:
  - Colonoscopy + gastroscopy
  - Iron studies
  - CT abdomen if colonoscopy normal
- **Pearl**: Unexplained iron-deficiency anemia in older men/postmenopausal women = **GI malignancy until ruled out**
- **Pitfall**: Simply giving iron supplements without investigating source

- 5. Change In Bowel Habits With Blood And Weight Loss

Case 5: The Constipated Retiree

Scenario: *A 67-year-old man reports increasing constipation, thinner stools, and occasional rectal bleeding over the last 3 months.*

He has also lost 4 kg unintentionally.

- **Red Flag**: New-onset change in bowel habits + rectal bleeding + weight loss
- **Differential Diagnosis**:
  - **Colorectal carcinoma**
  - Inflammatory bowel disease
  - Large polyps
  - Chronic constipation with fissures (less likely)
- **Next Steps**:
  - Colonoscopy
  - CEA (tumor marker)
  - Biopsy and staging CT if mass found
- **Pearl**: Blood mixed with stool and change in bowel habit in elderly = suspect **left-sided colon cancer**
- **Pitfall**: Attributing it to hemorrhoids without examining or investigating

- 6. Severe Abdominal Pain Out Of Proportion To Exam

Case 6: The Diabetic in Pain

Scenario: *A 72-year-old diabetic man presents with sudden severe abdominal pain but only mild tenderness on examination.*

He's in AF with a HR of 120.

- **Red Flag**: Pain out of proportion + AF + elderly
- **Diagnosis: Mesenteric ischemia**
- **Differential Diagnosis**:
    - Bowel obstruction
    - Perforated ulcer
    - Pancreatitis
- **Next Steps**:
    - Lactate, ABG (check for metabolic acidosis)
    - CT angiography of mesenteric vessels
    - Urgent surgical consult
- **Pearl**: Mesenteric ischemia often presents with **minimal signs early but rapid deterioration**
- **Pitfall**: Normal exam falsely reassuring early in ischemia

- 7. Recurrent Vomiting + Abdominal Distension

Case 7: The Obstructed Abdomen

Scenario: *A 60-year-old woman with history of abdominal surgery presents with vomiting, colicky abdominal pain, and bloating.*

No flatus or bowel movements in 2 days.

- **Red Flag**: No bowel movement + vomiting + previous surgery
- **Diagnosis**: **Small bowel obstruction** (likely adhesions)
- **Differential Diagnosis**:
  - Large bowel obstruction
  - Ileus
  - Volvulus
- **Next Steps**:
  - Abdominal X-ray (air-fluid levels)
  - CT abdomen and pelvis
  - NPO, NG tube, IV fluids
  - Surgical referral
- **Pearl**: Adhesions are the most common cause of **small bowel obstruction** in patients with prior surgery
- **Pitfall**: Giving oral fluids/meds before ruling out obstruction

- 8. Bloody Diarrhea + Fever + Tachycardia

Case 8: The Toxic Colon

Scenario: *A 35-year-old man with ulcerative colitis presents with severe bloody diarrhea, abdominal distension, fever, and tachycardia. WBCs and CRP are elevated.*

- **Red Flag**: Bloody diarrhea + systemic features + distension
- **Diagnosis: Toxic megacolon**
- **Differential Diagnosis**:
    - Infectious colitis
    - Ischemic colitis
    - Crohn's disease flare
- **Next Steps**:
    - Abdominal X-ray (check for colonic dilation >6 cm)
    - NPO, IV steroids, fluids
    - Surgical consult
- **Pearl**: A distended abdomen in IBD = rule out **toxic megacolon**
- **Pitfall**: Giving antidiarrheals in this setting can worsen condition

PAEDIATRICS: RED FLAGS

- 1. Failure To Thrive (Ftt)

Case 1: The Undergrowing Infant

Scenario: *A 4-month-old infant presents with poor weight gain. He was born at term with a birth weight of 3.2 kg but now weighs only 4.2 kg.*

Mum reports frequent feeding but persistent vomiting and loose stools.

- **Red Flags**: Crossing percentiles downward, persistent vomiting, poor feeding
- **Differential Diagnosis**:
  - Congenital heart disease
  - Malabsorption (e.g., coeliac disease, cystic fibrosis)
  - Neglect or poor feeding technique
  - Gastroesophageal reflux disease (GORD)
- **Next Steps**:
  - Full growth chart review (weight, length, head circumference)
  - Thorough feeding and social history
  - Screen for infections, cardiac murmur, stool studies
  - Nutritional support and consider admission
- **Pearl**: Failure to thrive can be **medical, nutritional, or social**—take a broad view
- **Pitfall**: Assuming it's always due to parental neglect without full workup

- 2. Bulging Fontanelle + Fever

Case 2: The Irritable Baby

Scenario: *A 9-month-old presents with fever, irritability, and vomiting.*

On exam, the anterior fontanelle is bulging. Neck stiffness is difficult to assess.

- **Red Flags**: Bulging fontanelle, irritability, vomiting
- **Differential Diagnosis**:
    - **Meningitis**
    - Encephalitis
    - Hydrocephalus
    - Intracranial hemorrhage
- **Next Steps**:
    - Immediate IV access, blood cultures
    - Urgent lumbar puncture (unless contraindicated)
    - Start empirical IV antibiotics (e.g., ceftriaxone) and antivirals (acyclovir)
- **Pearl**: In infants, **meningitis signs can be subtle**—fontanelle bulge is key
- **Pitfall**: Delaying treatment for lumbar puncture results—**treat first**

- 3. Persistent Vomiting In A Neonate

Case 3: The Hungry Vomiter

Scenario: *A 3-week-old male baby presents with projectile vomiting after every feed.*

Parents report he is still hungry after vomiting and is losing weight.

- **Red Flags**: Projectile vomiting + weight loss in neonate
- **Diagnosis**: **Hypertrophic pyloric stenosis**
- **Differential Diagnosis**:
  - GERD
  - Gastroenteritis
  - Intestinal obstruction
- **Next Steps**:
  - Check for palpable "olive" in RUQ
  - Ultrasound abdomen (confirm pyloric stenosis)
  - Correct dehydration/metabolic alkalosis
  - Surgical referral for pyloromyotomy
- **Pearl**: Pyloric stenosis classically presents at **2–6 weeks**, more common in boys
- **Pitfall**: Dismissing as reflux without checking hydration and growth

- 4. Delayed Milestones

Case 4: The Quiet Toddler

Scenario: *A 2-year-old boy is brought in for a routine check. He doesn't speak any clear words, doesn't make eye contact, and still walks with a wide, unsteady gait.*

No concerns in pregnancy or birth history.

- **Red Flags**: No words at 2 years, poor eye contact, motor delay
- **Differential Diagnosis**:
  - **Autism spectrum disorder**
  - Global developmental delay
  - Cerebral palsy
  - Hearing impairment

- **Next Steps**:
  - Formal developmental screening (Denver, ASQ)
  - Hearing and vision testing
  - Paediatric neurology and early intervention referral
  - Screen for metabolic/genetic conditions
- **Pearl**: Always **compare milestones** across all domains —motor, language, social
- **Pitfall**: Reassuring parents without investigating— **early intervention is key**

- 5. Petechiae And Bruising

Case 5: The Spotty Child

Scenario: *A 5-year-old child presents with fever, lethargy, and a new widespread petechial rash that does not blanch.*

He is drowsy and has cold peripheries.

- **Red Flags**: Non-blanching rash + fever + altered mental state
- **Differential Diagnosis**:
  - **Meningococcal septicaemia**
  - Immune thrombocytopenia
  - Leukemia
  - HSP (Henoch-Schönlein purpura)
- **Next Steps**:
  - Emergency antibiotics (ceftriaxone)
  - IV fluids, blood cultures, FBC, clotting
  - Transfer to PICU if unstable
- **Pearl**: A petechial rash with fever is **meningococcal until proven otherwise**

- **Pitfall**: Waiting for labs or LP before starting antibiotics

- 6. Limping Child + Refusal To Walk

Case 6: The Quiet Limp

Scenario: *A 4-year-old girl presents with refusal to walk and hip pain. No trauma reported.*

She had a cold last week. She is afebrile and otherwise well.

- **Red Flags:** Limp + refusal to weight bear
- **Differential Diagnosis:**
  - **Septic arthritis**
  - Transient synovitis
  - Legg-Calvé-Perthes disease
  - Leukemia
- **Next Steps:**
  - ESR, CRP, blood culture
  - X-ray pelvis and hips
  - Consider urgent ultrasound and orthopaedic consult
  - Joint aspiration if septic arthritis suspected
- **Pearl**: Any child refusing to walk **needs urgent evaluation**
- **Pitfall**: Attributing limp to "growing pains" or viral illness without ruling out serious causes

- 7. Seizure In A Child >5 Without Fever

Case 7: The New Fit

Scenario: *A 6-year-old boy presents with a generalized tonic-clonic seizure lasting 3 minutes.*

He had no fever. Parents report no previous seizures.

- **Red Flags**: First seizure >5 years old, no fever
- **Differential Diagnosis**:
    - **Epilepsy**
    - Space-occupying lesion
    - Head trauma
    - Metabolic derangement
- **Next Steps**:
    - Blood sugar, electrolytes, calcium
    - Neuro exam
    - EEG and brain MRI
    - Neurology referral
- **Pearl**: Febrile seizures usually occur **between 6 months and 5 years**
- **Pitfall**: Labelling as "febrile seizure" inappropriately and delaying neuro referral

- 8. Persistent Abdominal Pain With Weight Loss

Case 8: The Skinny Teen

Scenario: *A 12-year-old boy presents with 3 months of intermittent abdominal pain, diarrhea, and weight loss.*

He also reports fatigue and mouth ulcers.

- **Red Flags**: Chronic pain + diarrhea + weight loss + extra-GI symptoms
- **Differential Diagnosis**:
  - **Crohn's disease**
  - Coeliac disease
  - Juvenile IBD
  - Parasitic infection
- **Next Steps**:
  - FBC, CRP, ESR, iron studies
  - Stool calprotectin
  - Refer to paediatric gastroenterology
  - Endoscopy and biopsy
- **Pearl**: Chronic GI symptoms + weight loss = **always investigate for IBD**
- **Pitfall**: Mislabeling as "IBS" in children or ignoring growth faltering

DERMATOLOGY: RED FLAGS

- 1. Rapidly Growing Pigmented Lesion

Case 1: The Changing Mole

Scenario: *A 45-year-old woman presents with a mole on her upper back that has changed in size and color over the past 2 months.*

She also reports occasional itching and bleeding.

- **Red Flags**: Change in size, shape, color; bleeding; itching
- **Differential Diagnosis**:
  - **Melanoma**
  - Dysplastic nevus
  - Seborrheic keratosis
  - Pigmented basal cell carcinoma
- **Next Steps**:
  - Use **ABCDE** criteria (Asymmetry, Border, Color, Diameter >6mm, Evolution)
  - Urgent dermatology referral
  - Excisional biopsy with narrow margins
- **Pearl**: Any **changing pigmented lesion** = suspect melanoma
- **Pitfall**: Freezing or shaving suspicious lesions without biopsy

- 2. Blistering Rash In Older Adult

Case 2: The Blistered Back

Scenario: *A 72-year-old man presents with itchy, tense blisters on his lower abdomen and groin for 1 week.*

No mucosal involvement. No new medications.

- **Red Flags**: Blistering in elderly, pruritus, negative Nikolsky sign
- **Differential Diagnosis**:
  - **Bullous pemphigoid**
  - Pemphigus vulgaris
  - Dermatitis herpetiformis
  - Drug eruption
- **Next Steps**:
  - Skin biopsy for H&E and direct immunofluorescence
  - Start oral corticosteroids if confirmed
  - Consider dermatology referral
- **Pearl**: **Bullous pemphigoid** = elderly + tense blisters + no mucosal involvement
- **Pitfall**: Confusing it with contact dermatitis or shingles

- 3. Purple, Net-Like Rash On Legs

Case 3: The Lacy Legs

Scenario: *A 28-year-old woman presents with a lacy, violaceous rash on her lower legs.*

She also reports joint pain and mouth ulcers.

- **Red Flags**: Livedo reticularis + systemic symptoms (arthralgia, ulcers)
- **Differential Diagnosis**:
  - **Vasculitis** (e.g., SLE, PAN)
  - Antiphospholipid syndrome

- Cryoglobulinemia
- Cholesterol emboli
- **Next Steps**:
  - ANA, ENA, anti-dsDNA, antiphospholipid antibodies
  - FBC, ESR, CRP
  - Rheumatology referral
- **Pearl**: **Livedo reticularis** can be a cutaneous sign of systemic autoimmune disease
- **Pitfall**: Ignoring the skin as a clue to serious internal pathology

- 4. Painful Skin With Crepitus Or Bullae

Case 4: The Angry Leg

Scenario: *A 60-year-old diabetic man presents with severe pain in his left leg, redness, and swelling.*

The skin is discolored with blistering, and there's a crackling sound under the skin on palpation.

- **Red Flags**: Pain out of proportion, rapid progression, crepitus
- **Diagnosis**: **Necrotizing fasciitis**
- **Differential Diagnosis**:
  - Cellulitis
  - DVT
  - Gas gangrene
- **Next Steps**:
  - Urgent surgical referral
  - Broad-spectrum IV antibiotics (e.g., meropenem + clindamycin)
  - ICU care
- **Pearl**: **Pain > appearance = red flag** for necrotizing fasciitis
- **Pitfall**: Treating with oral antibiotics and discharging —**can be fatal**

- 5. New-Onset Rash + Systemic Symptoms After Drug

Case 5: The Rashy Reaction

Scenario: *A 35-year-old woman presents with fever, malaise, facial edema, and a widespread maculopapular rash.*

She started allopurinol 3 weeks ago.

- **Red Flags**: Rash + fever + eosinophilia + facial edema
- **Diagnosis**: **DRESS syndrome (Drug Reaction with Eosinophilia and Systemic Symptoms)**
- **Differential Diagnosis**:
    - SJS/TEN
    - Viral exanthem
    - Scarlet fever
- **Next Steps**:
    - Stop the offending drug immediately
    - CBC, LFTs, renal function, eosinophils
    - Hospital admission ± steroids
- **Pearl: DRESS can occur 2–6 weeks after drug initiation**
- **Pitfall**: Dismissing it as viral exanthem or allergy

- 6. Non-Healing Ulcer On Sun-Exposed Area

Case 6: The Lingering Lesion

Scenario: *A 68-year-old man presents with a non-healing ulcer on his cheek.*

It has been slowly enlarging over 3 months. He has a history of heavy sun exposure.

- **Red Flags**: Chronic ulceration, rolled border, sun-exposed location
- **Differential Diagnosis**:
  - **Basal cell carcinoma (BCC)**
  - Squamous cell carcinoma (SCC)
  - Keratoacanthoma
  - Chronic infection
- **Next Steps**:
  - Full skin exam
  - Biopsy for histology
  - Surgical excision or Mohs surgery
- **Pearl: Any lesion not healing in 6–8 weeks must be biopsied**
- **Pitfall**: Treating repeatedly as bacterial/fungal infection

- 7. Purpura In Febrile Child

Case 7: The Purple Child

Scenario: *A 3-year-old presents with high fever, vomiting, and a purpuric rash over the trunk and limbs.*

The child is lethargic and tachycardic.

- **Red Flags**: Fever + purpura + lethargy
- **Differential Diagnosis**:
  - **Meningococcaemia**
  - Sepsis
  - ITP
  - DIC
- **Next Steps**:
  - Immediate IV ceftriaxone
  - IV fluids, full septic screen
  - PICU referral
- **Pearl**: **Non-blanching rash + fever = medical emergency**
- **Pitfall**: Waiting for confirmation before antibiotics

- 8. Target Lesions And Mucosal Involvement

Case 8: The Red Mouth

Scenario: *A 19-year-old male presents with painful targetoid skin lesions, lip crusting, and conjunctival redness.*

He recently had a sore throat treated with antibiotics.

- **Red Flags**: Target lesions + mucosal involvement
- **Diagnosis**: **Stevens-Johnson Syndrome (SJS)**
- **Differential Diagnosis**:
  - Erythema multiforme
  - Toxic epidermal necrolysis (TEN)
  - Viral exanthem
- **Next Steps**:
  - Stop all suspected drugs
  - Admit to burns/dermatology unit
  - Supportive care ± IVIG or steroids
- **Pearl**: SJS is usually triggered by drugs (e.g., sulfa, anticonvulsants)
- **Pitfall**: Not recognizing early mucosal signs

ORTHOPAEDICS: RED FLAGS

- 1. Acute Back Pain With Neurological Deficit

Case 1: The Numb Legs

Scenario: *A 42-year-old man presents with severe lower back pain after lifting a heavy box.*

He reports bilateral leg weakness, numbness in the saddle area, and difficulty passing urine.

- **Red Flags**:
    - Saddle anaesthesia
    - Bladder/bowel dysfunction
    - Bilateral leg weakness
- **Differential Diagnosis**:
    - **Cauda equina syndrome**
    - Massive central disc herniation
    - Spinal abscess
    - Spinal trauma
- **Next Steps**:
    - Immediate **MRI lumbosacral spine**
    - Urgent neurosurgical/spinal referral
    - Do **not delay** for conservative management
- **Pearl: Cauda equina = surgical emergency**
- **Pitfall**: Sending home with analgesia without rectal or neuro exam

- 2. Red, Hot, Swollen Joint With Fever

Case 2: The Angry Knee

Scenario: *A 65-year-old diabetic man presents with a painful, swollen, red left knee.*

He is febrile and cannot bear weight.

- **Red Flags**:
  - Fever
  - Monoarthritis
  - Rapid joint destruction
  - Systemic symptoms
- **Differential Diagnosis**:
  - **Septic arthritis**
  - Crystal arthropathy
  - Inflammatory arthritis
  - Reactive arthritis
- **Next Steps**:
  - Joint aspiration (send for Gram stain, culture, crystals, WCC)
  - Blood cultures
  - IV antibiotics immediately after aspiration
  - Orthopaedic referral for possible washout
- **Pearl: Septic arthritis can destroy joint in hours**
- **Pitfall**: Assuming it's gout in a patient with fever and not aspirating

- 3. Long Bone Pain In A Child

Case 3: The Limping Boy

Scenario: *A 9-year-old boy presents with a limp and left thigh pain for 2 weeks. No trauma.*

On exam, he has point tenderness over the femur and a low-grade fever.

- **Red Flags**:
  - Bone pain, especially at night
  - Fever
  - Limp without trauma
  - Systemic symptoms
- **Differential Diagnosis**:
  - **Osteomyelitis**
  - Ewing's sarcoma
  - Bone cyst
  - Growing pains (less likely)
- **Next Steps**:
  - CBC, ESR, CRP
  - MRI of femur
  - Blood cultures
  - Paediatric orthopaedic referral
- **Pearl: Persistent bone pain in kids = rule out malignancy/infection**
- **Pitfall**: Dismissing as growing pains without investigating

- 4. Back Pain + Weight Loss + Night Sweats

Case 4: The Hidden Spine Problem

Scenario: *A 67-year-old man presents with chronic lower back pain, night sweats, and unintentional weight loss.*

He has a history of smoking.

- **Red Flags**:

- ◦ Night pain
- ◦ Weight loss
- ◦ History of malignancy
- ◦ Neurological symptoms
- **Differential Diagnosis**:
  - ◦ **Spinal metastasis** (prostate, lung, breast, kidney)
  - ◦ Multiple myeloma
  - ◦ Spinal TB
  - ◦ Discitis
- **Next Steps**:
  - ◦ X-ray spine, ESR/CRP, PSA
  - ◦ MRI whole spine
  - ◦ Urgent referral to oncology/orthopaedics
- **Pearl**: **Back pain with systemic symptoms needs urgent imaging**
- **Pitfall**: Treating as mechanical pain in an elderly patient without red flag screening

- 5. Sudden Leg Pain Post-Hip Surgery

Case 5: The Cold Leg

Scenario: *A 75-year-old woman post-total hip replacement complains of severe left leg pain and coldness.*

The foot is pale and pulseless.

- **Red Flags**:
  - ◦ Sudden onset severe limb pain
  - ◦ Pallor, pulselessness, paraesthesia
  - ◦ Post-operative context
- **Diagnosis**: **Acute limb ischaemia**

- **Differential Diagnosis**:
  - Arterial embolism
  - DVT (less likely to cause pulselessness)
  - Compartment syndrome (tense calf)
- **Next Steps**:
  - Urgent vascular referral
  - Doppler US or CT angiography
  - Anticoagulation, possibly embolectomy
- **Pearl**: **Post-op vascular events need fast recognition to save limb**
- **Pitfall**: Confusing with DVT or neuropathy

- 6. Swollen Leg After Fracture

Case 6: The Tight Calf

Scenario: *A 28-year-old male with a mid-shaft tibia fracture in a cast presents with increasing pain, swelling, and numbness in the toes.*

- **Red Flags**:
  - Pain out of proportion
  - Pain on passive stretch
  - Tense compartment
  - Paraesthesia, pallor
- **Diagnosis: Acute compartment syndrome**
- **Next Steps**:
  - Remove cast immediately
  - Check compartment pressures if in doubt
  - Emergency fasciotomy
- **Pearl: 6 Ps: Pain, Pallor, Pulselessness, Paraesthesia, Paralysis, Pressure**
- **Pitfall**: Delaying recognition—**this is a true**

orthopaedic emergency

- 7. Painless Lump In Long Bone

Case 7: The Silent Tumour

Scenario: *A 19-year-old male notices a painless swelling over his distal femur.*

It has been slowly growing over months. No systemic symptoms.

- **Red Flags**:
    - Painless enlarging mass
    - Young age
    - Long bone location
    - No history of trauma
- **Differential Diagnosis**:
    - **Osteosarcoma**
    - Ewing sarcoma
    - Benign bone cyst
    - Osteochondroma
- **Next Steps**:
    - Plain X-ray
    - MRI with contrast
    - Refer urgently to sarcoma unit
- **Pearl**: **Any painless bone lump = rule out primary bone malignancy**
- **Pitfall**: Assuming it's a sports injury or benign lump

- 8. Chronic Shoulder Pain In Diabetic

Case 8: The Frozen Shoulder

Scenario: *A 56-year-old woman with poorly controlled diabetes complains of a stiff, painful shoulder worsening over months,* *especially with movement.*

- **Red Flags**:
  - Progressive stiffness
  - Limited passive and active movement
  - Functional limitation
- **Diagnosis: Adhesive capsulitis (Frozen shoulder)**
- **Next Steps**:
  - Rule out red flags like rotator cuff tear or tumour
  - Imaging if uncertain
  - Physiotherapy and steroid injections
- **Pearl: Frozen shoulder is common in diabetics and thyroid disease**
- **Pitfall**: Overlooking treatable causes like rotator cuff tears

NEPHROLOGY: RED FLAGS

- 1. Rapidly Rising Creatinine With Systemic Symptoms

Case 1: The Failing Kidneys

Scenario: *A 55-year-old man presents with malaise, dark urine, joint pain, and a new purpuric rash.*

His creatinine has risen from 90 to 300 μmol/L in 3 weeks. Urinalysis shows blood and protein.

- **Red Flags**:
    - Rapid decline in renal function
    - Haematuria + proteinuria
    - Systemic symptoms (fever, rash, arthralgia)
    - New-onset hypertension
- **Differential Diagnosis**:
    - **Rapidly progressive glomerulonephritis (RPGN)**
    - ANCA-associated vasculitis
    - Lupus nephritis
    - Post-infectious GN
- **Next Steps**:
    - Urine microscopy, U&E, ANCA, ANA, anti-dsDNA, complement levels
    - Urgent **renal biopsy**
    - Start steroids +/- immunosuppressants after biopsy
- **Pearl: RPGN = kidney emergency; can lead to ESRD in**

weeks if untreated
- **Pitfall**: Delaying nephrology referral for biopsy

- 2. Anuria Or Oliguria With Volume Overload

Case 2: The Swollen Man

Scenario: *A 64-year-old hypertensive diabetic man presents with shortness of breath, swollen legs, and has not passed urine for 2 days. Crackles in both lung bases and JVP is elevated.*

- **Red Flags**:
  - Anuria/oliguria
  - Pulmonary oedema
  - Rising creatinine
  - Hyperkalaemia
- **Differential Diagnosis**:
  - **Acute kidney injury (AKI)** — pre-renal, renal, post-renal
  - Obstructive uropathy
  - Cardiorenal syndrome
- **Next Steps**:
  - Check catheter for output
  - Bedside bladder scan
  - U&E, ABG, ECG (for potassium)
  - Urgent dialysis if refractory pulmonary oedema or severe hyperkalaemia
- **Pearl: AKI + pulmonary oedema not responding to diuretics → consider urgent dialysis**
- **Pitfall**: Overhydration in oliguric patients

- 3. Severe Hyperkalaemia (K+ >6.5 Mmol/L)

Case 3: The Peaked T Waves

Scenario: *A 70-year-old man with CKD stage 4 presents after missing dialysis.*

ECG shows tall peaked T waves, bradycardia, and a wide QRS.

- **Red Flags**:
  - Potassium >6.5 mmol/L
  - ECG changes
  - Muscle weakness or arrhythmias
  - Missed dialysis sessions
- **Differential Diagnosis**:
  - CKD or ESRD
  - Medications (ACEi, ARBs, spironolactone)
  - Adrenal insufficiency
- **Next Steps**:
  - **IV calcium gluconate** for cardiac membrane stabilization
  - **IV insulin + glucose**
  - Salbutamol nebulisers, sodium bicarbonate (if acidotic)
  - Urgent dialysis if refractory
- **Pearl: Treat ECG, not just lab values in hyperkalaemia**
- **Pitfall**: Delaying dialysis in the presence of cardiac toxicity

- 4. Gross Haematuria With Proteinuria

Case 4: The Cola-Coloured Urine

Scenario: *A 23-year-old man presents with cola-coloured urine after a sore throat 2 weeks ago.*

Urinalysis shows 3+ blood and 2+ protein.

- **Red Flags**:

- ◦ Gross or persistent microscopic haematuria
- ◦ Proteinuria (>1g/day)
- ◦ Recent infection
- ◦ Hypertension
- **Differential Diagnosis**:
  - ◦ **Post-streptococcal glomerulonephritis**
  - ◦ IgA nephropathy
  - ◦ Lupus nephritis
  - ◦ Thin basement membrane disease
- **Next Steps**:
  - ◦ Urine microscopy and protein/creatinine ratio
  - ◦ ASO titre, complement levels
  - ◦ Monitor renal function
  - ◦ Nephrology referral if renal function deteriorates or nephrotic range proteinuria
- **Pearl: Dark urine post-infection → think glomerular cause, not UTI**
- **Pitfall**: Misdiagnosing as UTI or ignoring significant proteinuria

- 5. Nephrotic Syndrome In A Young Adult

Case 5: The Puffy Eyes

Scenario: *A 25-year-old male presents with facial puffiness, scrotal swelling, and frothy urine.*

BP is 140/90. Urine shows 4+ protein, no blood.

- **Red Flags**:
  - ◦ Edema (especially periorbital)
  - ◦ Proteinuria >3.5g/day
  - ◦ Hypoalbuminaemia

- Hyperlipidaemia
- **Differential Diagnosis**:
  - **Minimal change disease**
  - Focal segmental glomerulosclerosis (FSGS)
  - Membranous nephropathy
  - Secondary causes: SLE, infections, malignancy
- **Next Steps**:
  - 24h urine protein or spot protein/creatinine ratio
  - Serum albumin, lipids
  - ANA, HIV, Hep B/C serologies
  - Renal biopsy in adults
- **Pearl: Adult nephrotic syndrome always needs biopsy to determine cause**
- **Pitfall**: Starting steroids before confirming diagnosis

- 6. Polyuria With Severe Thirst

Case 6: The Constantly Drinking Man

Scenario: *A 34-year-old man reports urinating 10–12 times a day with constant thirst.*

Serum Na+ is 150 mmol/L. Glucose is normal. Urine osmolality is low.

- **Red Flags**:
  - Polyuria + polydipsia
  - High-normal or high sodium
  - Low urine osmolality
- **Differential Diagnosis**:
  - **Diabetes insipidus**
  - Psychogenic polydipsia

- Osmotic diuresis (less likely)
- **Next Steps**:
  - Water deprivation test
  - Desmopressin trial
  - Serum and urine osmolality
- **Pearl**: **Polyuria + dilute urine + high sodium = suspect DI**
- **Pitfall**: Assuming diabetes mellitus in every polyuric patient

- 7. Hypertension In A Young Adult With Low K+

Case 7: The Resistant BP

Scenario: *A 29-year-old woman with resistant hypertension and persistent hypokalaemia presents for evaluation.*

No history of diuretics.

- **Red Flags**:
  - Resistant hypertension
  - Hypokalaemia
  - Young age
  - No secondary cause found
- **Differential Diagnosis**:
  - **Primary hyperaldosteronism (Conn's syndrome)**
  - Renal artery stenosis
  - Cushing's syndrome
  - Liddle syndrome
- **Next Steps**:
  - Plasma aldosterone/renin ratio
  - 24h urinary potassium

- ○ Adrenal CT if positive
- ○ Refer to endocrinology/nephrology
- · **Pearl: Young + HTN + low K = think secondary cause**
- · **Pitfall**: Treating with multiple antihypertensives without investigating cause

- 8. Sudden Bilateral Flank Pain And Haematuria

Case 8: The Bleeding Kidneys

Scenario: *A 48-year-old man with known autosomal dominant polycystic kidney disease (ADPKD) presents with flank pain and visible haematuria after mild trauma.*

- · **Red Flags**:
  - ○ Known ADPKD
  - ○ Gross haematuria
  - ○ Flank mass
  - ○ Family history of renal failure
- · **Differential Diagnosis**:
  - ○ Cyst rupture or bleeding
  - ○ Nephrolithiasis
  - ○ Pyelonephritis
  - ○ Renal tumour
- · **Next Steps**:
  - ○ Non-contrast CT KUB
  - ○ Monitor haemoglobin
  - ○ Pain control, hydration
  - ○ Nephrology follow-up
- · **Pearl: ADPKD can cause spontaneous cyst rupture/ bleeding**

- **Pitfall**: Dismissing haematuria as minor in a known cystic kidney

ENDOCRINOLOGY: RED FLAGS

- 1. Hyperthyroidism With Tremor, Weight Loss, And Tachycardia

Case 1: The Agitated Patient

Scenario: *A 45-year-old woman presents with recent unintentional weight loss (5 kg in 2 weeks), tremors, palpitations, and feeling overly warm despite normal temperatures.*

On examination, she has a fine tremor, tachycardia (110 bpm), and a soft goiter.

- **Red Flags**:
    - Unexplained weight loss
    - Tachycardia, palpitations
    - Tremor, heat intolerance
    - Soft, diffuse goiter
- **Differential Diagnosis**:
    - **Graves' disease**
    - Toxic multinodular goiter
    - Thyroid storm (if severely symptomatic)
    - Subacute thyroiditis
- **Next Steps**:
    - Serum TSH, free T4, and free T3
    - Thyroid antibody testing (TRAb)
    - Neck ultrasound if goiter is present
    - **Consider radioactive iodine uptake scan** (if indicated)
- **Pearl: Graves' disease is the most common cause of**

hyperthyroidism in younger women.

- **Pitfall**: Confusing hyperthyroidism with anxiety or menopause

- 2. Hypothyroidism With Weight Gain And Fatigue

Case 2: The Tired and Slow Patient

Scenario: *A 60-year-old woman presents with complaints of fatigue, weight gain (despite no change in diet), constipation, dry skin, and hair thinning.*

On examination, her pulse is slow, and her reflexes are delayed. She has a goiter.

- **Red Flags**:
    - Weight gain without dietary changes
    - Fatigue, cold intolerance
    - Dry skin, hair thinning
    - Bradycardia, delayed reflexes
    - Goiter
- **Differential Diagnosis**:
    - **Hashimoto's thyroiditis** (most common cause of hypothyroidism)
    - Iodine deficiency
    - Pituitary or hypothalamic dysfunction
    - Drug-induced (e.g., lithium)
- **Next Steps**:
    - Serum TSH, free T4
    - Thyroid antibodies (anti-TPO, anti-thyroglobulin)
    - Consider ultrasound of the thyroid if a goiter is present

- **Pearl**: **In elderly patients, hypothyroidism may present as depression or cognitive decline**
- **Pitfall**: Overlooking the possibility of hypothyroidism in an elderly patient with vague symptoms

- 3. Adrenal Insufficiency With Hypotension And Hyperpigmentation

Case 3: The Tired, Tan Patient

Scenario: *A 39-year-old woman with a history of autoimmune disease presents with progressive fatigue, dizziness upon standing, and darkening of her skin, especially around the neck and armpits.*

She reports weight loss, nausea, and loss of appetite.

- **Red Flags**:
    - Chronic fatigue
    - Orthostatic hypotension
    - Hyperpigmentation (especially in sun-exposed areas)
    - GI symptoms (nausea, weight loss, anorexia)
- **Differential Diagnosis**:
    - **Addison's disease** (primary adrenal insufficiency)
    - Secondary adrenal insufficiency (due to pituitary or hypothalamic dysfunction)
    - Chronic use of steroids
- **Next Steps**:
    - Serum cortisol, ACTH
    - Morning cortisol (before 9 AM)
    - ACTH stimulation test

- Electrolytes (look for hyponatremia, hyperkalemia)
- Chest imaging if tuberculosis or metastasis is suspected

- **Pearl: Hyperpigmentation in Addison's disease is due to increased ACTH, which shares a precursor with melanocyte-stimulating hormone (MSH).**
- **Pitfall**: Missing adrenal insufficiency in patients with vague complaints like fatigue or anorexia

- 4. Hypercalcemia With Polyuria And Polydipsia

Case 4: The Thirsty, Urinating Patient

Scenario: *A 50-year-old man presents with excessive thirst, frequent urination, and confusion. He also reports nausea, constipation, and general weakness.*

Blood tests show a calcium level of 12 mg/dL (normal 8.5–10.5 mg/ dL).

- **Red Flags**:
  - Hypercalcemia (elevated calcium level)
  - Polyuria, polydipsia
  - Confusion, weakness
  - Gastrointestinal symptoms (nausea, constipation)
- **Differential Diagnosis**:
  - **Primary hyperparathyroidism**
  - Malignancy (e.g., multiple myeloma, lung cancer)
  - Granulomatous disease (e.g., sarcoidosis, tuberculosis)
  - Vitamin D toxicity
- **Next Steps**:

- Parathyroid hormone (PTH) level
- PTH-related peptide (PTHrP)
- 25-hydroxyvitamin D level
- Consider imaging for malignancy (CXR, bone scan)
  - **Pearl**: **Primary hyperparathyroidism is the most common cause of hypercalcemia.**
  - **Pitfall**: Misdiagnosing hypercalcemia as dehydration or renal failure

- 5. Cushing's Syndrome With Weight Gain And Purple Striae

Case 5: The Moon Faced Patient

Scenario: *A 45-year-old woman presents with recent weight gain, particularly in her abdomen and face. She also reports easy bruising, purple striae on her abdomen, and thinning skin.*

She has a history of long-term corticosteroid use for asthma.

- **Red Flags**:
  - Central obesity, moon face, buffalo hump
  - Purple striae, easy bruising
  - Skin thinning
  - History of chronic steroid use
- **Differential Diagnosis**:
  - **Cushing's disease** (ACTH-secreting pituitary adenoma)
  - **Ectopic ACTH syndrome** (e.g., lung carcinoma)
  - **Iatrogenic Cushing's** (due to corticosteroid use)
- **Next Steps**:

- Serum cortisol (midnight, or 24-hour urinary free cortisol)
- ACTH level (to differentiate between adrenal, pituitary, and ectopic causes)
- Dexamethasone suppression test
- MRI pituitary for suspected Cushing's disease
- **Pearl: Iatrogenic Cushing's syndrome is common in patients on long-term steroids.**
- **Pitfall**: Failing to consider iatrogenic causes when a patient on steroids presents with features of Cushing's syndrome

- 6. Diabetes Mellitus With Weight Loss And Polyuria

Case 6: The Thin, Thirsty Patient

Scenario: *A 30-year-old woman with a family history of diabetes presents with excessive thirst, frequent urination, and unintentional weight loss.*

Her blood glucose is 400 mg/dL, and HbA1c is 11%.

- **Red Flags**:
    - Polyuria, polydipsia
    - Weight loss despite increased appetite
    - Elevated blood glucose
    - Family history of diabetes
- **Differential Diagnosis**:
    - **Type 1 diabetes mellitus** (more common in

younger individuals)

- **Type 2 diabetes mellitus**
- **Diabetic ketoacidosis (DKA)** (if acidosis is present)

- **Next Steps**:
  - Urinalysis for ketones (check for DKA)
  - C-peptide level (to differentiate between Type 1 and Type 2)
  - Diabetic education and initiation of insulin therapy if Type 1
  - Consider screening for other autoimmune conditions (e.g., thyroid disease, celiac disease)

- **Pearl**: **Unintentional weight loss despite a good appetite is a hallmark of Type 1 diabetes.**

- **Pitfall**: Delaying the diagnosis of Type 1 diabetes in adults due to the assumption that diabetes is always Type 2

- 7. Hypoglycemia With Sweating And Tremor

Case 7: The Fainting Diabetic

Scenario: *A 60-year-old diabetic man on insulin presents with a history of recent episodes of sweating, shaking, and confusion, especially in the early morning.*

His blood sugar at the time of one episode was 40 mg/dL.

- **Red Flags**:
  - Hypoglycemia (blood sugar <70 mg/dL)
  - Sweating, tremor, confusion
  - Recent changes in diet or exercise routine
  - Use of insulin or sulfonylureas

- **Differential Diagnosis**:

- ○ **Insulin-induced hypoglycemia**
- ○ **Sulfonylurea-induced hypoglycemia**
- ○ **Addison's disease** (adrenal insufficiency)
- ○ **Insulinoma** (rare)
- **Next Steps**:
  - ○ Check blood glucose levels during episodes
  - ○ Review medication regimen (including insulin doses)
  - ○ 72-hour fast if insulinoma is suspected
  - ○ Consider checking cortisol levels if Addison's disease is suspected
- **Pearl: Patients on insulin may experience hypoglycemia even with minor changes in diet or exercise.**
- **Pitfall**: Misdiagnosing hypoglycemia in patients with other symptoms (e.g., confusion from other causes)

RHEUMATOLOGY: RED FLAGS

- 1. Rheumatoid Arthritis With Joint Swelling And Morning Stiffness

Case 1: The Stiff and Swollen Hands

Scenario: *A 40-year-old woman presents with a 2-month history of bilateral swelling and pain in her wrists, MCP joints, and knees.*

She reports morning stiffness lasting 1-2 hours and has difficulty with daily tasks like brushing her hair and opening jars. She has a family history of rheumatoid arthritis.

- **Red Flags**:
  - Bilateral joint swelling (particularly small joints)
  - Morning stiffness >30 minutes
  - Symmetrical involvement
  - Difficulty with activities of daily living (e.g., grip strength loss)
  - Family history of rheumatoid arthritis
- **Differential Diagnosis**:
  - **Rheumatoid arthritis (RA)**
  - Psoriatic arthritis
  - Osteoarthritis
  - Systemic lupus erythematosus (SLE)
- **Next Steps**:
  - Rheumatoid factor (RF) and anti-CCP antibodies

- ° X-rays of affected joints
- ° ESR and CRP for inflammation
- ° Joint aspiration if joint effusion is present (for crystal analysis)
- **Pearl: Early treatment of RA with DMARDs (e.g., methotrexate) can prevent long-term joint damage.**
- **Pitfall**: Misdiagnosing RA as osteoarthritis or assuming only elderly individuals get RA

- 2. Systemic Lupus Erythematosus (Sle) With Butterfly Rash And Photosensitivity

Case 2: The Butterfly Rash

Scenario: *A 32-year-old woman presents with a butterfly-shaped rash across her cheeks and nose, along with joint pain in her hands and wrists.*

She reports fatigue, photosensitivity, and recent hair thinning. She has a history of recurrent oral ulcers and feels generally unwell.

- **Red Flags**:
  - ° Butterfly-shaped facial rash (malar rash)
  - ° Photosensitivity
  - ° Oral ulcers
  - ° Joint pain (arthralgia)
  - ° Fatigue, hair thinning
- **Differential Diagnosis**:
  - ° **Systemic lupus erythematosus (SLE)**
  - ° Dermatomyositis
  - ° Psoriatic arthritis
  - ° Drug-induced lupus (e.g., hydralazine, procainamide)

- **Next Steps**:
    - ANA (antinuclear antibody) testing
    - Anti-dsDNA and anti-Smith antibodies (specific for SLE)
    - Urinalysis (for proteinuria or hematuria, as kidney involvement is common)
    - ESR and CRP to assess disease activity
- **Pearl: SLE can affect multiple organ systems, so a multi-disciplinary approach is often required.**
- **Pitfall**: Overlooking SLE in young women with vague symptoms like fatigue and joint pain

- 3. Gout With Acute Joint Pain And Redness

Case 3: The Painful, Red Toe

Scenario: *A 55-year-old man with a history of hypertension and hyperlipidemia presents with sudden, severe pain and redness in his right big toe.*

He mentions consuming a large amount of seafood and alcohol over the weekend.

On examination, the joint is erythematous, swollen, and extremely tender to touch.

- **Red Flags**:
    - Acute, severe joint pain (typically at night)
    - Redness, swelling, and tenderness in a single joint (especially the first MTP joint)
    - History of high purine intake (alcohol, seafood)
    - Known risk factors for hyperuricemia (e.g., obesity, hypertension)
- **Differential Diagnosis**:
    - **Gout** (acute gouty arthritis)
    - Pseudogout
    - Septic arthritis
    - Trauma or fracture
- **Next Steps**:
    - Joint aspiration and synovial fluid analysis for urate crystals
    - Serum uric acid (although may not be elevated during acute attacks)
    - X-ray to rule out joint damage or other causes

- ESR and CRP for inflammation
- **Pearl**: **Gout commonly affects the first MTP joint and can often be triggered by dietary factors.**
- **Pitfall**: Failing to aspirate the joint during an acute attack and misdiagnosing as other causes of arthritis

- 4. Ankylosing Spondylitis With Morning Back Pain And Stiffness

Case 4: The Stiff, Young Man

Scenario: *A 28-year-old man presents with chronic low back pain and stiffness that worsens in the morning and improves with activity.*

He has a history of heel pain (Achilles tendinitis) and reports difficulty bending his back. His father has ankylosing spondylitis.

- **Red Flags**:
    - Chronic back pain and stiffness (especially in younger patients <40 years)
    - Pain improves with exercise, worsens at rest
    - Peripheral involvement (e.g., Achilles tendinitis, hip pain)
    - Family history of ankylosing spondylitis
- **Differential Diagnosis**:
    - **Ankylosing spondylitis (AS)**
    - Psoriatic arthritis
    - Osteoarthritis of the spine
    - Reactive arthritis
- **Next Steps**:
    - HLA-B27 testing (genetic marker)
    - X-rays of the sacroiliac joints (for early changes of AS)

- ESR and CRP for inflammation
  - MRI if suspected early-stage sacroiliitis
- **Pearl**: **Ankylosing spondylitis may present with extra-articular manifestations, including uveitis.**
- **Pitfall**: Delayed diagnosis due to misinterpretation of early back pain as mechanical or non-specific

- 5. Scleroderma With Skin Thickening And Raynaud's Phenomenon

Case 5: The Tight-Skinned Patient

Scenario: *A 50-year-old woman presents with complaints of tight skin on her hands and face, along with difficulty opening her mouth.*

She also mentions experiencing episodes of cold-induced color changes in her fingers (Raynaud's phenomenon), which turn white and then blue in cold weather.

- **Red Flags**:
  - Skin thickening and tightening (particularly on hands and face)
  - Difficulty with mouth opening (due to skin tightness)
  - Raynaud's phenomenon (color changes in fingers)
  - GERD (gastroesophageal reflux disease) or swallowing difficulties
- **Differential Diagnosis**:
  - **Systemic sclerosis (scleroderma)**
  - Localized scleroderma
  - Lupus erythematosus

- ◦ Dermatomyositis
- . **Next Steps**:
  - ◦ ANA testing (most patients with scleroderma are ANA positive)
  - ◦ Anti-centromere antibodies (associated with limited systemic sclerosis)
  - ◦ Anti-Scl-70 antibodies (associated with diffuse systemic sclerosis)
  - ◦ Nailfold capillaroscopy to assess for vascular changes
- . **Pearl: Scleroderma can cause significant morbidity due to internal organ involvement (e.g., lungs, heart, kidneys).**
- . **Pitfall**: Confusing limited scleroderma with Raynaud's phenomenon alone

- 6. Polymyositis/Dermatomyositis With Muscle Weakness And Skin Rash

Case 6: The Weak and Rashy Patient

Scenario: *A 40-year-old woman presents with progressive muscle weakness, especially in the shoulders and hips, making it difficult for her to rise from a seated position or climb stairs.*

She also has a heliotrope rash (purple rash around her eyes) and Gottron's papules (raised red bumps over the knuckles).

- . **Red Flags**:
  - ◦ Progressive muscle weakness (especially in proximal muscles)
  - ◦ Heliotrope rash (around eyes)
  - ◦ Gottron's papules (on knuckles)
  - ◦ Difficulty rising from a chair or combing hair

- **Differential Diagnosis**:
  - **Polymyositis**
  - **Dermatomyositis**
  - Inclusion body myositis
  - Hypothyroid myopathy
- **Next Steps**:
  - Creatine kinase (CK) and aldolase (markers of muscle damage)
  - Muscle biopsy (for definitive diagnosis)
  - ANA testing (to look for underlying autoimmune etiology)
  - EMG (electromyography) to assess for muscle involvement
- **Pearl: Dermatomyositis can involve the skin, muscles, and even the lungs (interstitial lung disease).**
- **Pitfall**: Delaying diagnosis in patients with insidious onset of muscle weakness and subtle skin findings

NEUROLOGY2: RED FLAGS

- 1. Acute Stroke With Sudden Onset Of Weakness And Speech Difficulty

Case 1: The Sudden Loss of Speech and Strength

Scenario: *A 68-year-old man with a history of hypertension presents to the ER with sudden-onset right-sided weakness and inability to speak clearly.*

He also has difficulty understanding what people are saying. The symptoms began 1 hour ago while he was watching TV.

- **Red Flags**:
  - Sudden-onset unilateral weakness (hemiparesis)
  - Sudden-onset speech difficulties (aphasia or dysarthria)
  - Hemisensory loss
  - Sudden loss of vision or double vision
- **Differential Diagnosis**:
  - **Ischemic stroke**
  - Hemorrhagic stroke
  - Transient ischemic attack (TIA)
  - Brain tumor or mass effect
- **Next Steps**:
  - Immediate CT scan of the brain to rule out hemorrhage
  - MRI for more detailed assessment of ischemic

areas

- National Institutes of Health Stroke Scale (NIHSS) for assessing severity
- Blood glucose (to rule out hypoglycemia)
- Initiate thrombolysis or thrombectomy if within therapeutic window (ischemic stroke)

- **Pearl: Time is brain—stroke treatment is time-sensitive, and early intervention can significantly reduce morbidity.**
- **Pitfall**: Delaying neuroimaging in patients with subtle symptoms, leading to a missed diagnosis of stroke.

- 2. Meningitis With Fever, Neck Stiffness, And Photophobia

Case 2: The Feverish, Stiff Neck

Scenario: *A 25-year-old man presents with a 2-day history of fever, severe headache, and a stiff neck.*

He also reports sensitivity to light and nausea. On examination, he has a positive Brudzinski sign and a fever of 39°C.

- **Red Flags**:
  - Sudden-onset fever and severe headache
  - Neck stiffness (positive Brudzinski or Kernig signs)
  - Photophobia and nausea
  - Altered mental status or confusion
- **Differential Diagnosis**:
  - **Bacterial meningitis**
  - Viral meningitis
  - Fungal meningitis

- ◦ Subarachnoid hemorrhage
- **Next Steps**:
    - ◦ Lumbar puncture (LP) for cerebrospinal fluid (CSF) analysis
    - ◦ Blood cultures and CBC for infection markers
    - ◦ CT scan of the head (to rule out mass effect or hemorrhage before LP)
    - ◦ Empirical antibiotics (including ceftriaxone and vancomycin) pending culture results
- **Pearl**: **Bacterial meningitis requires immediate empirical treatment with antibiotics and corticosteroids to reduce mortality.**
- **Pitfall**: Delaying lumbar puncture in suspected bacterial meningitis due to fear of herniation. Always perform a CT scan first if there are concerns.

- 3. Seizures With Loss Of Consciousness And Tonic-Clonic Movements

Case 3: The Seizing Patient

Scenario: *A 35-year-old woman presents with a witnessed episode of generalized tonic-clonic seizures.*

The episode lasted for 2 minutes, followed by confusion and drowsiness.

There is no previous history of seizures or head trauma. Her medical history is unremarkable, but she is under stress due to work pressures.

- **Red Flags**:
    - ◦ Sudden, witnessed loss of consciousness
    - ◦ Generalized tonic-clonic movements
    - ◦ Postictal confusion or drowsiness

○ No previous history of seizures

- **Differential Diagnosis**:
  - ○ **Epileptic seizure (focal or generalized)**
  - ○ Syncope (especially if with a preceding prodrome)
  - ○ Non-epileptic attack disorder (psychogenic)
  - ○ Hypoglycemia, hyponatremia, or electrolyte disturbances

- **Next Steps**:
  - ○ EEG to confirm seizure activity (if persistent concerns for epilepsy)
  - ○ MRI or CT scan of the brain to rule out structural lesions (e.g., tumors, vascular malformations)
  - ○ Electrolyte panel, glucose, and liver function tests
  - ○ Consider starting antiepileptic drugs if epilepsy is suspected

- **Pearl: The postictal state (confusion or sleepiness) can last for minutes to hours, and recovery can vary depending on seizure duration and etiology.**

- **Pitfall**: Misdiagnosing a seizure as syncope without proper evaluation of the postictal state and EEG findings.

- 4. Multiple Sclerosis With Visual Changes And Limb Weakness

Case 4: The Young Woman with Vision and Coordination Issues

Scenario: *A 29-year-old woman presents with a 2-week history of worsening vision in her right eye, associated with numbness and weakness in her left leg.*

She reports occasional double vision and difficulty walking. She denies any trauma.

On examination, she has an impaired visual acuity in the right eye and a positive Romberg test.

- **Red Flags:**
  - Visual disturbances (e.g., optic neuritis, diplopia)
  - Limb weakness or numbness (especially if asymmetrical)
  - Difficulty with coordination or balance (ataxia)
  - Young woman, typically age 20-40 years
- **Differential Diagnosis:**
  - **Multiple sclerosis (MS)**
  - Neuromyelitis optica
  - Transverse myelitis
  - Optic neuritis due to other causes (e.g., infection, sarcoidosis)
- **Next Steps:**
  - MRI of the brain and spinal cord with contrast to look for plaques of demyelination
  - Lumbar puncture (CSF analysis for oligoclonal bands)
  - Visual evoked potentials (VEP) for optic nerve involvement
- **Pearl: Multiple sclerosis is often relapsing-remitting, and treatment with disease-modifying therapies (DMTs) can help manage relapses.**
- **Pitfall:** Missing the diagnosis of MS in patients with a "flare-up" that is misattributed to a viral illness or stress.

- 5. Parkinson's Disease With Resting Tremor And Bradykinesia

Case 5: The Shaky, Slowed Movements

Scenario: *A 65-year-old man presents with a 6-month history of a resting tremor in his right hand, which is noticeable at rest and improves with movement.*

He also complains of stiffness, especially in the mornings, and has noticed slowness in his gait.

He has difficulty getting out of chairs and has a slight stooped posture.

- **Red Flags**:
    - Resting tremor (often unilateral)
    - Bradykinesia (slowness of movement)
    - Muscle rigidity (cogwheel rigidity)
    - Gait changes (shuffling steps, decreased arm swing)
- **Differential Diagnosis**:
    - **Parkinson's disease (PD)**
    - Essential tremor
    - Drug-induced parkinsonism (e.g., antipsychotics)
    - Wilson's disease (especially in younger patients)
- **Next Steps**:
    - Clinical diagnosis based on motor symptoms (the "TRAP" mnemonic: tremor, rigidity, akinesia, postural instability)
    - MRI brain (to rule out secondary causes of parkinsonism, such as stroke or tumor)

- Dopamine transporter (DAT) scan for atypical cases or diagnostic uncertainty
  - **Pearl**: **Parkinson's disease is a progressive neurodegenerative disorder that can be managed with dopaminergic medications (e.g., levodopa) and lifestyle interventions.**
  - **Pitfall**: Overlooking early signs of Parkinson's disease in elderly patients who may attribute symptoms to normal aging.

- 6. Myasthenia Gravis With Muscle Weakness And Fatigue

Case 6: The Patient with Fatigue and Weakness

Scenario: *A 45-year-old woman presents with complaints of progressively worsening muscle weakness over the past month.*

She reports difficulty swallowing, drooping eyelids (ptosis), and double vision, especially later in the day. Symptoms improve with rest.

She denies any past medical history of similar symptoms.

- **Red Flags**:
  - Muscle weakness that worsens with activity and improves with rest
  - Ptosis and/or diplopia (ocular symptoms)
  - Difficulty swallowing or speaking (bulbar symptoms)
  - Young or middle-aged woman, often in the setting of autoimmune disease
- **Differential Diagnosis**:
  - **Myasthenia gravis (MG)**

- ◦ Lambert-Eaton syndrome
- ◦ Guillain-Barré syndrome (GBS)
- ◦ Stroke (but usually with more focal findings)
- **Next Steps**:
  - ◦ Serum acetylcholine receptor antibodies (AChR Ab)
  - ◦ Edrophonium test (Tensilon test)
  - ◦ Electrodiagnostic testing (repetitive nerve stimulation)
  - ◦ CT or MRI chest to look for thymoma
- **Pearl: Myasthenia gravis can cause both ocular and bulbar symptoms, and treatment includes anticholinesterase medications and immunosuppressants.**
- **Pitfall**: Delaying diagnosis or attributing symptoms to stress or general weakness, missing the opportunity for early intervention.

PSYCHIATRY: RED FLAGS

- 1. Major Depressive Disorder With Suicidal Thoughts

Case 1: The Depressed Patient with Suicidal Ideation

Scenario: *A 35-year-old woman presents to the emergency department with a 2-week history of low mood, lack of energy, and loss of interest in activities she once enjoyed.*

She also reports poor sleep, significant weight loss, and frequent thoughts of death.

She says she has been thinking about ending her life but hasn't made any plans.

- **Red Flags**:
    - Persistent low mood for more than 2 weeks
    - Loss of interest or pleasure in previously enjoyed activities (anhedonia)
    - Significant weight loss or changes in appetite
    - Suicidal thoughts or ideation (especially without a safety plan)
    - Sleep disturbances (insomnia or hypersomnia)
    - Feelings of worthlessness or guilt
- **Differential Diagnosis**:
    - **Major depressive disorder (MDD)**
    - Bipolar disorder (depressive episode)

- ○ Generalized anxiety disorder (GAD)
- ○ Adjustment disorder with depressed mood
- ○ Substance-induced mood disorder (e.g., alcohol or drug abuse)
- **Next Steps**:
  - ○ Immediate risk assessment for suicidal ideation, intent, and plan
  - ○ Hospitalization if the patient is at high risk for suicide
  - ○ Mental state examination (MSE) and thorough history
  - ○ Consider starting an antidepressant (e.g., SSRI) and psychotherapy (e.g., CBT)
  - ○ Establish a safety plan and provide emergency contacts
- **Pearl: Suicidal ideation in major depression requires urgent intervention, including both pharmacological and psychotherapeutic approaches.**
- **Pitfall**: Minimizing the risk of suicide in patients who are not immediately vocal about their plans—always assess the severity of suicidal ideation carefully.

- 2. Acute Psychosis With Hallucinations And Delusions

Case 2: The Young Man with Hearing Voices

Scenario: *A 22-year-old male presents with a 3-day history of hearing voices that are not there, which have been telling him that people are plotting against him.*

He believes that he is being watched and followed by the government. He is visibly agitated and paranoid.

His history is significant for substance use, but he denies recent drug use.

- **Red Flags**:
    - Acute onset of hallucinations (auditory, visual, or tactile)
    - Delusions (paranoid, persecutory, or grandiose)
    - Disorganized thinking or speech
    - Severe agitation or violence
    - Abrupt change in behavior or functioning
- **Differential Diagnosis**:
    - **Schizophrenia**
    - Substance-induced psychosis (e.g., drugs, alcohol)
    - Brief psychotic disorder
    - Delusional disorder
    - Bipolar disorder (mania with psychotic features)
    - Organic causes (e.g., infection, brain tumor)
- **Next Steps**:
    - Immediate psychiatric evaluation and mental state examination (MSE)
    - Urine toxicology screening to rule out substance-induced causes
    - Brain imaging (CT or MRI) to rule out organic causes
    - Initiate antipsychotic medication (e.g., haloperidol, olanzapine)
    - Consider hospitalization if there is risk to self or others
- **Pearl**: **A thorough evaluation is required to distinguish between primary psychotic disorders**

and secondary causes like substance use or medical conditions.

- **Pitfall**: Failing to rule out organic causes (e.g., encephalitis, brain injury) in patients with sudden-onset psychosis.

- 3. Generalized Anxiety Disorder (Gad) With Excessive Worry

Case 3: The Woman Who Can't Stop Worrying

Scenario: *A 40-year-old woman presents with excessive worry about her health, finances, and her children, which she says has been going on for the past 6 months.*

She finds it difficult to control the worry, and it interferes with her daily activities.

She also reports restlessness, muscle tension, and trouble concentrating.

- **Red Flags**:
  - Excessive and uncontrollable worry lasting for more than 6 months
  - Physical symptoms like muscle tension, restlessness, and irritability
  - Difficulty concentrating or mind going blank
  - Sleep disturbances (insomnia or hypersomnia)
  - Impaired functioning (e.g., work, social)
- **Differential Diagnosis**:
  - **Generalized anxiety disorder (GAD)**
  - Panic disorder
  - Social anxiety disorder
  - Adjustment disorder with anxiety
  - Thyroid disorder (e.g., hyperthyroidism)
- **Next Steps**:
  - Screen for GAD using self-report questionnaires (e.g., GAD-7)

- Consider ruling out medical causes (e.g., thyroid function tests, CBC)
- Start a course of cognitive behavioral therapy (CBT)
- Pharmacotherapy options (e.g., SSRIs like sertraline)
- Teach relaxation techniques and stress management strategies

- **Pearl: In GAD, the worry is often disproportionate to the actual threat and can lead to significant impairment in daily life. Therapy is effective in managing symptoms.**

- **Pitfall**: Overlooking the physical symptoms (muscle tension, sleep disturbances) that are common in anxiety disorders, and misdiagnosing them as purely physical conditions.

- 4. Bipolar Disorder With Manic Episode

Case 4: The Man with Elevated Mood and Impulsivity

Scenario: *A 30-year-old man presents with a 2-week history of increased energy, racing thoughts, and excessive spending.*

He reports sleeping only 3-4 hours a night and feeling "on top of the world."

He has been overly talkative and has been making impulsive decisions, such as quitting his job and buying a new car he cannot afford.

- **Red Flags:**

- Elevated or irritable mood for at least 1 week
- Increased energy and decreased need for sleep
- Impulsivity (e.g., excessive spending, reckless behavior)
- Grandiosity or inflated self-esteem
- Racing thoughts or pressured speech

- **Differential Diagnosis**:
  - **Bipolar disorder (mania)**
  - Substance-induced mood disorder (e.g., stimulants, alcohol)
  - Schizophrenia (mania with psychotic features)
  - Hyperthyroidism
  - Attention-deficit hyperactivity disorder (ADHD)

- **Next Steps**:
  - Mental state examination to assess for manic symptoms
  - Screen for substance use disorders (e.g., urine toxicology)
  - Start mood stabilizers (e.g., lithium, valproate)
  - Consider antipsychotic medication if psychotic features are present (e.g., quetiapine)
  - Assess for risk of harm (e.g., self-harm or harm to others)

- **Pearl: Mania is a psychiatric emergency if there is risk of harm to self or others. Hospitalization may be required in severe cases.**

- **Pitfall**: Misdiagnosing mania as generalized excitement or normal behavior, which can delay treatment and result in further impairment.

- 5. Post-Traumatic Stress Disorder (Ptsd) With Intrusive Thoughts

Case 5: The Veteran with Flashbacks and Hypervigilance

Scenario: *A 40-year-old male veteran presents with nightmares, intrusive memories, and flashbacks of his combat experiences.*

He reports that he avoids crowds, is constantly on edge, and has difficulty trusting others.

He is irritable and has trouble sleeping.

- **Red Flags**:
    - Recurrent, intrusive memories or flashbacks of a traumatic event
    - Hypervigilance or exaggerated startle response
    - Emotional numbing or avoidance of trauma reminders
    - Sleep disturbances (nightmares, insomnia)
    - Negative alterations in mood or cognition
- **Differential Diagnosis**:
    - **Post-traumatic stress disorder (PTSD)**
    - Acute stress disorder
    - Adjustment disorder
    - Panic disorder
    - Depression with trauma-related symptoms

- **Next Steps**:
    - Screen for PTSD using self-report questionnaires (e.g., PTSD Checklist—PCL-5)
    - Trauma-focused cognitive behavioral therapy (CBT)
    - Eye movement desensitization and reprocessing (EMDR)
    - Pharmacotherapy (e.g., SSRIs such as sertraline)
- **Pearl: PTSD requires trauma-focused therapy and often medication to reduce intrusive symptoms. Early intervention is key to preventing chronicity.**
- **Pitfall**: Failing to consider PTSD in patients with trauma histories who present with nonspecific symptoms like irritability, sleep disturbance, or avoidance.

SURGERY: RED FLAGS

- 1. Acute Appendicitis

Case 1: The Young Patient with Abdominal Pain

Scenario: *A 24-year-old male presents with a 24-hour history of worsening abdominal pain, which started around the umbilicus and has now localized to the right lower quadrant.*

He also reports nausea, loss of appetite, and a mild fever (38°C).

On examination, he has localized tenderness and guarding in the right lower quadrant.

- **Red Flags:**
  - Abdominal pain migrating from the umbilical region to the right lower quadrant
  - Fever, nausea, and loss of appetite
  - Localized tenderness or guarding over the right iliac fossa
  - Positive rebound tenderness and/or Rovsing's sign
  - Elevated white blood cell count (leukocytosis)
- **Differential Diagnosis:**
  - **Acute appendicitis**
  - Ectopic pregnancy (in females)
  - Ovarian torsion (in females)
  - Inflammatory bowel disease (e.g., Crohn's disease)
  - Gastroenteritis or food poisoning

- **Next Steps**:
  - Clinical examination and lab tests (CBC with differential)
  - Consider imaging (e.g., abdominal ultrasound, CT scan)
  - If confirmed, surgical consultation for appendectomy
  - Prepare for urgent appendectomy if there is evidence of perforation or abscess formation
- **Pearl**: **The clinical diagnosis of appendicitis is often made on the basis of history and physical examination, but imaging (CT or ultrasound) is useful when the diagnosis is unclear.**
- **Pitfall**: Delaying surgical consultation or misdiagnosing appendicitis as other conditions (e.g., gastroenteritis), especially in younger patients.

- 2. Bowel Obstruction

Case 2: The Elderly Patient with Abdominal Distension

Scenario: *An 80-year-old female presents with a 2-day history of abdominal distension, cramping pain, and vomiting.*

She has been unable to pass stool or flatus. Her medical history includes previous abdominal surgeries, and she is currently on pain medications.

- **Red Flags**:
  - Abdominal distension, pain, and vomiting
  - Inability to pass stool or gas (constipation)
  - History of prior abdominal surgery (adhesions)
  - Dehydration (dry mucous membranes, tachycardia)
  - High-pitched bowel sounds or absence of bowel sounds
- **Differential Diagnosis**:
  - **Bowel obstruction** (mechanical, functional)
  - Adhesions or hernia (from prior surgery)
  - Volvulus (torsion of the bowel)
  - Intussusception (more common in children but can occur in adults)
  - Peritonitis
- **Next Steps**:
  - Abdominal X-ray to look for signs of bowel obstruction (dilated loops of bowel, air-fluid levels)
  - CT scan if diagnosis remains unclear

- Nasogastric tube for decompression and fluid resuscitation
- Surgical consultation for possible laparotomy if the obstruction is mechanical or there are signs of bowel ischemia

- **Pearl**: **Early recognition and management are key in preventing bowel ischemia or perforation in cases of bowel obstruction.**

- **Pitfall**: Misdiagnosing bowel obstruction as simple constipation, leading to delays in appropriate imaging and surgical consultation.

- 3. Gallbladder Disease (Cholecystitis Or Cholelithiasis)

Case 3: The Middle-Aged Woman with Right Upper Quadrant Pain

Scenario: *A 45-year-old woman presents with a 12-hour history of severe right upper quadrant abdominal pain, which started after a fatty meal.*

She also reports nausea and vomiting. On examination, she has tenderness over the right upper quadrant with a positive Murphy's sign.

- **Red Flags**:
    - Severe right upper quadrant pain, often triggered by a fatty meal
    - Nausea and vomiting
    - Fever and leukocytosis
    - Positive Murphy's sign (increased pain on inspiration while palpating the right

subcostal area)
- Jaundice (in case of choledocholithiasis)
- **Differential Diagnosis**:
  - **Acute cholecystitis** (inflammation of the gallbladder)
  - Cholelithiasis (gallstones)
  - Acute pancreatitis
  - Peptic ulcer disease or perforation
  - Hepatitis or liver abscess
- **Next Steps**:
  - Perform liver function tests (LFTs) and CBC
  - Abdominal ultrasound to detect gallstones and signs of cholecystitis
  - If confirmed, surgical consultation for cholecystectomy
  - Consider nonoperative management (e.g., antibiotics and IV fluids) if the patient is not a surgical candidate, but surgery is the definitive treatment
- **Pearl**: **Early surgical intervention is recommended for acute cholecystitis to avoid complications like gallbladder perforation or sepsis.**
- **Pitfall**: Failing to differentiate between simple gallstone pain (biliary colic) and acute cholecystitis, leading to delays in management.

- 4. Abdominal Aortic Aneurysm (Aaa)

Case 4: The Elderly Male with Severe Abdominal Pain

Scenario: *A 72-year-old male with a history of hypertension presents with sudden-onset severe lower abdominal pain that radiates to his* *back.*

He feels lightheaded and has a drop in blood pressure. He is at increased risk due to his smoking history.

- **Red Flags:**
    - Sudden-onset severe abdominal pain, often described as "tearing" or "ripping"
    - Radiating pain to the back
    - Hypotension or shock (tachycardia, diaphoresis)
    - Pulsatile mass in the abdomen (palpable in some cases)
    - History of hypertension, smoking, or family history of AAA
- **Differential Diagnosis:**
    - **Abdominal aortic aneurysm (AAA)** rupture
    - Acute pancreatitis
    - Mesenteric ischemia
    - Gastrointestinal perforation
    - Renal colic
- **Next Steps:**
    - Immediate abdominal ultrasound or CT scan to confirm the diagnosis
    - If AAA rupture is confirmed, urgent surgical intervention required (open or endovascular repair)
    - Resuscitate with IV fluids and blood products as necessary
    - Pain control and stabilization before surgery
- **Pearl: A ruptured AAA is a life-threatening emergency requiring immediate surgical**

intervention. **Rapid diagnosis and resuscitation are critical.**

- **Pitfall**: Misdiagnosing AAA rupture as less severe abdominal pain, delaying imaging and life-saving surgery.

- 5. Perforated Bowel (E.g., Perforated Peptic Ulcer)

Case 5: The Patient with Acute Abdominal Pain and Rigidity

Scenario: *A 55-year-old male with a history of chronic NSAID use presents with sudden-onset severe abdominal pain.*

On examination, he has diffuse tenderness and rigidity, with absent bowel sounds. He reports a history of peptic ulcer disease but has not been compliant with treatment.

- **Red Flags**:
    - Sudden-onset severe abdominal pain
    - Diffuse tenderness and abdominal rigidity (peritonitis)
    - Absent bowel sounds (paralytic ileus)
    - Fever and leukocytosis
    - History of peptic ulcer disease or chronic NSAID use
- **Differential Diagnosis**:
    - **Perforated peptic ulcer**
    - Bowel perforation from diverticulitis
    - Acute pancreatitis with retroperitoneal perforation
    - Mesenteric ischemia
    - Intestinal obstruction or ischemia
- **Next Steps**:

- Immediate abdominal X-ray to look for free air under the diaphragm (indicative of perforation)
- CT scan if necessary for further evaluation
- Surgical consultation for emergency laparotomy or laparoscopy
- Initiate IV antibiotics and resuscitation

- **Pearl**: **Perforation of a peptic ulcer is a surgical emergency. Early intervention can prevent sepsis and multi-organ failure.**
- **Pitfall**: Delaying surgery in patients with signs of peritonitis due to misdiagnosing them with less severe conditions like gastroenteritis.

LABORATORY MEDICINE: RED FLAGS

- 1. Anemia With Low Hemoglobin And Mcv

Case 1: The Elderly Female with Fatigue

Scenario: *A 70-year-old female presents with a 2-month history of fatigue, pallor, and occasional shortness of breath.*

She also reports a decrease in appetite and occasional dizziness. Blood tests reveal a hemoglobin of 9 g/dL, MCV of 70 fL, and a reticulocyte count of 1%.

- **Red Flags**:
    - Fatigue, pallor, and dizziness
    - Low hemoglobin and low MCV (microcytic anemia)
    - Reticulocyte count of 1% (suggesting a low bone marrow response)
- **Differential Diagnosis**:
    - **Iron deficiency anemia** (most common cause of microcytic anemia)
    - Anemia of chronic disease (due to underlying inflammatory conditions, cancer, or chronic infection)
    - Thalassemia (especially in populations of Mediterranean, Asian, or African descent)
    - Lead poisoning (less common, but possible)
- **Next Steps**:

- Iron studies (serum iron, ferritin, total iron-binding capacity) to confirm iron deficiency
- Consider stool occult blood test to rule out gastrointestinal bleeding
- Perform a peripheral blood smear to assess for anisocytosis or microcytosis
- Assess for underlying causes such as GI tract malignancy or chronic blood loss

- **Pearl: In elderly patients, microcytic anemia is often due to chronic disease or iron deficiency due to gastrointestinal blood loss. Careful workup is needed to rule out malignancy.**
- **Pitfall**: Misdiagnosing iron deficiency as anemia of chronic disease without confirming iron studies or a full workup.

- 2. Leukocytosis With Neutrophilia

Case 2: The Young Patient with Fever and Abdominal Pain

Scenario: *A 25-year-old male presents to the emergency department with a 1-day history of fever, abdominal pain, and nausea.*

His vital signs show a temperature of 38.5°C, heart rate of 110 bpm, and blood pressure of 125/80 mmHg.

A complete blood count (CBC) reveals a white blood cell count (WBC) of 18,000/μL with a neutrophil predominance (90%).

- **Red Flags**:
    - Fever and abdominal pain
    - Markedly elevated WBC count with neutrophil predominance
    - Tachycardia and fever
- **Differential Diagnosis**:
    - **Bacterial infection** (e.g., appendicitis, cholecystitis, diverticulitis, or pelvic inflammatory disease)
    - Sepsis (especially if there is organ dysfunction)
    - Inflammatory bowel disease (flare of Crohn's disease or ulcerative colitis)
    - Pyelonephritis or urinary tract infection (UTI)
- **Next Steps**:
    - Blood cultures and abdominal ultrasound to assess for appendicitis or cholecystitis
    - Urinalysis and urine culture to rule out UTI
    - CT scan of the abdomen and pelvis to identify inflammatory or infectious causes

- ◦ Initiate empirical broad-spectrum antibiotics pending culture results
- **Pearl: A neutrophil predominance in the presence of fever and abdominal pain suggests an ongoing bacterial infection, and the source must be identified and treated promptly.**
- **Pitfall**: Failing to consider non-infectious causes (e.g., inflammatory bowel disease) when neutrophilia is present, delaying proper management.

- 3. Thrombocytopenia With Bleeding Symptoms

Case 3: The Middle-Aged Male with Bruising

Scenario: *A 45-year-old male presents with a 1-week history of easy bruising, gingival bleeding, and petechial rash on his arms and legs. He denies any recent trauma.*

Blood tests show a platelet count of 30,000/μL, normal coagulation profile, and a normal hemoglobin level.

- **Red Flags**:
  - ◦ Easy bruising and gingival bleeding
  - ◦ Petechiae and purpura
  - ◦ Low platelet count (thrombocytopenia)
  - ◦ No history of trauma or anticoagulant use
- **Differential Diagnosis**:
  - ◦ **Idiopathic thrombocytopenic purpura (ITP)**
  - ◦ Acute leukemia (especially in adults)
  - ◦ Thrombotic thrombocytopenic purpura (TTP)
  - ◦ Disseminated intravascular coagulation (DIC)
  - ◦ Bone marrow failure (e.g., aplastic anemia or

myelodysplastic syndromes)

- **Next Steps**:
    - Peripheral blood smear to check for abnormal cells (e.g., blasts in leukemia, schistocytes in TTP)
    - Bone marrow biopsy if there is suspicion of marrow failure or leukemia
    - Evaluate for underlying causes (e.g., HIV, hepatitis, medications)
    - Platelet transfusion if bleeding is severe, and treatment based on diagnosis (e.g., corticosteroids for ITP)
- **Pearl: Thrombocytopenia with bleeding symptoms is a hematologic emergency and should prompt immediate workup to rule out life-threatening conditions like TTP or DIC.**
- **Pitfall**: Delaying diagnosis and treatment for serious conditions like TTP, especially when platelet counts are low but clinical features of hemolysis (e.g., jaundice) are present.

- 4. Hyperkalemia With Ecg Changes

Case 4: The Patient with Renal Failure and Electrolyte Imbalance

Scenario: *A 65-year-old male with a history of chronic kidney disease (CKD) and diabetes presents with weakness, nausea, and palpitations.*

His blood tests reveal a potassium level of 6.5 mmol/L. An ECG shows peaked T-waves and a prolonged QRS interval.

- **Red Flags**:
    - Elevated potassium (hyperkalemia)
    - ECG changes (peaked T-waves, prolonged QRS

interval)

- History of CKD or other risk factors for electrolyte imbalances

- **Differential Diagnosis**:
  - **Hyperkalemia** (due to impaired renal excretion or cellular release of potassium)
  - Renal failure (acute or chronic)
  - Medications (e.g., ACE inhibitors, potassium-sparing diuretics, NSAIDs)
  - Adrenal insufficiency (Addison's disease)
  - Hemolysis (artifact from improper blood sample handling)

- **Next Steps**:
  - Treat hyperkalemia immediately with calcium gluconate (to stabilize the myocardium), sodium bicarbonate, or insulin and glucose
  - Repeat potassium level to confirm and monitor trends
  - Review medication list to identify any drugs contributing to hyperkalemia
  - Initiate or adjust dialysis if the patient is anuric or in acute renal failure

- **Pearl**: **Hyperkalemia can be life-threatening, especially when there are ECG changes. Immediate intervention and monitoring are crucial to avoid fatal arrhythmias.**

- **Pitfall**: Failing to recognize the clinical significance of subtle ECG changes in hyperkalemia, especially in patients with renal dysfunction.

- 5. Liver Dysfunction With Jaundice

Case 5: The Alcoholic Patient with Jaundice

Scenario: *A 50-year-old male with a history of heavy alcohol use presents with yellowing of the skin and eyes, fatigue, and abdominal discomfort.*

His liver function tests (LFTs) reveal an AST of 350 U/L, ALT of 200 U/L, alkaline phosphatase of 150 U/L, and a total bilirubin of 5 mg/dL (with conjugated bilirubin being elevated).

- **Red Flags**:
    - Jaundice with elevated liver enzymes
    - Elevated bilirubin (especially conjugated)
    - History of alcohol use or liver disease
- **Differential Diagnosis**:
    - **Alcoholic liver disease (alcoholic hepatitis or cirrhosis)**
    - Viral hepatitis (e.g., hepatitis B, C)
    - Hepatic cirrhosis or fibrosis
    - Biliary obstruction (gallstones or malignancy)
    - Autoimmune hepatitis
- **Next Steps**:
    - Liver ultrasound to assess for liver cirrhosis or biliary obstruction
    - Hepatitis serologies (e.g., hepatitis B and C markers)
    - Consider liver biopsy or elastography for definitive diagnosis in cases of suspected cirrhosis
    - Abstinence from alcohol and supportive care for alcoholic hepatitis if diagnosed
- **Pearl: Jaundice with elevated AST and ALT, especially**

in the context of alcohol use, is a strong indicator of alcoholic liver disease, but other causes must be ruled out.

- **Pitfall**: Misattributing jaundice and liver enzyme abnormalities solely to alcohol use without further investigation, missing other treatable liver conditions.

OBSTETRICS: RED FLAGS

- 1. Severe Abdominal Pain With Vaginal Bleeding In Early Pregnancy

Case 1: The 28-Year-Old with Abdominal Pain

Scenario: *A 28-year-old woman at 7 weeks of gestation presents to the emergency department with severe lower abdominal pain and moderate vaginal bleeding.*

She reports a 3-day history of spotting, now with increasing pain and heavier bleeding. Ultrasound reveals a 5 cm mass in the left adnexa with no intrauterine pregnancy identified.

- **Red Flags**:
    - Severe abdominal pain and vaginal bleeding in early pregnancy
    - No intrauterine pregnancy seen on ultrasound
    - Presence of an adnexal mass
- **Differential Diagnosis**:
    - **Ectopic pregnancy** (most likely diagnosis in this case)
    - Spontaneous abortion (miscarriage)
    - Ovarian cyst rupture or torsion
    - Molar pregnancy
- **Next Steps**:
    - Serum beta-hCG to check for a rising or falling pattern (helpful for diagnosing ectopic

pregnancy)

- Transvaginal ultrasound to assess for ectopic pregnancy and further evaluate the adnexal mass
- Consultation with obstetrics and gynecology for possible laparoscopy or management of ectopic pregnancy
- Monitor blood loss and hemoglobin levels if hemorrhage is suspected

- **Pearl**: **Ectopic pregnancies are a life-threatening emergency and require prompt diagnosis and management to prevent rupture and hemorrhage.**
- **Pitfall**: Failing to consider ectopic pregnancy in patients with early pregnancy bleeding and abdominal pain, which can delay life-saving intervention.

- 2. Severe Hypertension With Proteinuria In Late Pregnancy

Case 2: The 32-Year-Old with Headaches and Swelling

Scenario: *A 32-year-old woman at 34 weeks gestation presents with complaints of headaches, visual disturbances, and swelling in her hands and feet.*

Her blood pressure is measured at 160/100 mmHg, and her urine dipstick shows +2 protein.

She is otherwise healthy, with no history of hypertension.

- **Red Flags**:
    - Severe hypertension (BP >140/90 mmHg) in pregnancy
    - Proteinuria (suggesting preeclampsia)
    - Symptoms of headaches and visual

disturbances (indicating possible cerebral involvement)

- **Differential Diagnosis**:
  - **Preeclampsia** (most likely diagnosis)
  - Chronic hypertension exacerbated by pregnancy
  - Gestational hypertension (without proteinuria or organ damage)
  - HELLP syndrome (hemolysis, elevated liver enzymes, low platelet count)
- **Next Steps**:
  - Confirm diagnosis of preeclampsia with a 24-hour urine collection for protein quantification
  - Assess for signs of HELLP syndrome (liver function tests, platelet count)
  - Hospital admission for close monitoring of blood pressure, urine output, and fetal wellbeing
  - Consider initiating antihypertensive therapy (e.g., labetalol) if BP remains elevated
  - Plan for delivery if severe features of preeclampsia are present (e.g., BP >160/110, thrombocytopenia, liver dysfunction)
- **Pearl**: **Preeclampsia is a leading cause of maternal morbidity and mortality. Timely diagnosis and management are crucial, with delivery being the only definitive treatment.**
- **Pitfall**: Failing to recognize the early signs of preeclampsia, especially in women without a history of hypertension, which can lead to delayed diagnosis and complications.

- 3. Sudden Loss Of Fetal Movement In Third Trimester

Case 3: The 30-Year-Old with Decreased Fetal Movement

Scenario: *A 30-year-old woman at 38 weeks of gestation presents with concerns about decreased fetal movement.*

She has noticed a marked reduction in movement over the past 12 hours. She has no pain, bleeding, or other symptoms.

Her pregnancy has been uncomplicated until now.

- **Red Flags**:
    - Decreased or absent fetal movement in the third trimester
    - No other symptoms (e.g., bleeding, cramping) to explain the change in fetal movement
- **Differential Diagnosis**:
    - **Fetal distress** (possible hypoxia or intrauterine growth restriction)
    - Oligohydramnios (low amniotic fluid volume)
    - Placental abruption
    - Umbilical cord accidents (e.g., cord prolapse, cord entanglement)
- **Next Steps**:
    - Non-stress test (NST) to evaluate fetal heart rate and movement
    - Ultrasound to assess amniotic fluid volume and fetal growth
    - Consider biophysical profile (BPP) for further fetal monitoring
    - If any concerns arise, consider delivery based on fetal well-being, gestational age, and

clinical situation

- **Pearl: Decreased fetal movement is often a sign of fetal distress, and prompt evaluation is necessary to ensure fetal well-being.**
- **Pitfall**: Delaying assessment and management, thinking that decreased fetal movement is a normal variation, which can lead to poor neonatal outcomes if fetal distress is not identified.

- 4. Heavy Vaginal Bleeding After Delivery (Postpartum Hemorrhage)

Case 4: The Postpartum Woman with Excessive Bleeding

Scenario: *A 25-year-old woman, 2 hours post vaginal delivery, presents with excessive vaginal bleeding.*

Her blood loss exceeds 500 mL within the first hour after delivery, and she complains of dizziness and lightheadedness.

Her pulse is 110 bpm, and her blood pressure is 90/60 mmHg.

- **Red Flags**:
  - Heavy vaginal bleeding (>500 mL after vaginal delivery, >1000 mL after cesarean section)
  - Hypotension and tachycardia (signs of shock)
  - Dizziness and lightheadedness (signs of blood loss)
- **Differential Diagnosis**:
  - **Postpartum hemorrhage (PPH)** due to uterine atony (most common cause)
  - Retained placenta or placental fragments
  - Lacerations or uterine rupture
  - Coagulopathy (e.g., disseminated

intravascular coagulation - DIC)

- **Next Steps**:
  - ○ Uterine massage and oxytocin administration to manage uterine atony
  - ○ Inspect for retained placenta or lacerations and repair as necessary
  - ○ Laboratory tests to assess hemoglobin, platelet count, and coagulation profile (e.g., fibrinogen levels)
  - ○ Consider uterine artery embolization or surgery (e.g., hysterectomy) if bleeding is uncontrolled
- **Pearl: Postpartum hemorrhage is a leading cause of maternal morbidity and mortality. Early intervention with uterine massage and medications like oxytocin can prevent further blood loss.**
- **Pitfall**: Underestimating blood loss and failing to act promptly, which can result in hypovolemic shock and increased maternal morbidity.

- 5. Severe Pelvic Pain With Fever And Malodorous Discharge

Case 5: The 27-Year-Old with Postpartum Fever

Scenario: *A 27-year-old woman presents with fever (38.5°C), severe lower abdominal pain, and foul-smelling vaginal discharge 5 days postpartum.*

She had a vaginal delivery with no complications.

Physical examination reveals uterine tenderness, and the cervix is slightly dilated with purulent discharge.

- **Red Flags**:
    - Fever and pelvic pain postpartum
    - Malodorous discharge and uterine tenderness
    - Postpartum period (5 days after delivery)
- **Differential Diagnosis**:
    - **Endometritis** (infection of the uterine lining, most commonly following cesarean or prolonged labor)
    - Pelvic inflammatory disease (PID)
    - Retained products of conception (which can lead to infection)
    - Urinary tract infection (UTI) or pyelonephritis
- **Next Steps**:
    - Blood cultures and vaginal swabs to identify the causative organism
    - Broad-spectrum intravenous antibiotics (e.g., ceftriaxone and metronidazole) until culture results are available
    - Consider ultrasound to rule out retained

products of conception

- Pain management and hydration

- **Pearl**: **Endometritis is a common postpartum infection, especially after cesarean delivery. Early identification and treatment with antibiotics can prevent complications like sepsis.**

- **Pitfall**: Failing to recognize the importance of thorough examination and early antibiotic therapy in postpartum women with fever and pelvic pain, which can lead to severe infection and sepsis.

GYNAECOLOGY: RED FLAGS

- 1. Postmenopausal Bleeding

Case 1: The 55-Year-Old with Bleeding

Scenario: *A 55-year-old woman, 3 years post-menopause, presents with a complaint of vaginal bleeding.*

She notes a small amount of blood on her underwear after urination and is concerned.

Her periods had stopped regularly after menopause, and she is otherwise healthy with no significant medical history.

- **Red Flags**:
  - Any vaginal bleeding after menopause (postmenopausal bleeding)
  - Recent cessation of periods with new onset of bleeding
- **Differential Diagnosis**:
  - **Endometrial carcinoma** (most concerning diagnosis for postmenopausal bleeding)
  - Endometrial hyperplasia
  - Uterine polyps
  - Vaginal atrophy (due to low estrogen)
  - Coagulopathies or bleeding disorders
- **Next Steps**:
  - Pelvic examination to assess the cervix and uterus

- Transvaginal ultrasound (TVUS) to measure endometrial thickness
- Endometrial biopsy if the endometrial lining is thickened or there is concern for malignancy
- Consider hysteroscopy for direct visualization and biopsy

- **Pearl**: **Postmenopausal bleeding should never be considered normal and warrants evaluation to rule out malignancy.**

- **Pitfall**: Assuming postmenopausal bleeding is always due to benign causes like vaginal atrophy, without ruling out more serious conditions like endometrial cancer.

- 2. Pelvic Pain With Dyspareunia And Menstrual Irregularities

Case 2: The 32-Year-Old with Pelvic Pain

Scenario: *A 32-year-old woman presents with pelvic pain, especially during intercourse (dyspareunia), and irregular menstrual cycles.*

She reports heavy periods with clotting and sometimes pain that lasts for several days.

She also complains of occasional back pain and bloating.

- **Red Flags**:
  - Chronic pelvic pain, especially with sexual intercourse (dyspareunia)
  - Menstrual irregularities, including heavy bleeding
  - Associated back pain and bloating
- **Differential Diagnosis**:

- **Endometriosis** (most likely diagnosis based on symptoms of pelvic pain and dyspareunia)
- Pelvic inflammatory disease (PID)
- Ovarian cysts
- Uterine fibroids
- Adenomyosis

- **Next Steps**:
  - Pelvic examination to check for masses, tenderness, or signs of infection
  - Transvaginal ultrasound to assess for fibroids, ovarian cysts, or other abnormalities
  - Laparoscopy for definitive diagnosis of endometriosis, especially if symptoms persist despite medical treatment
  - Consider laparoscopy or MRI for more detailed assessment in complex cases

- **Pearl**: **Endometriosis is a chronic, often underdiagnosed condition that can cause severe pelvic pain and infertility. Early diagnosis can improve quality of life.**

- **Pitfall**: Misdiagnosing endometriosis as IBS or pelvic inflammatory disease when the symptoms of chronic pelvic pain and menstruation-related discomfort persist.

- 3. Abnormal Vaginal Discharge With Odour

Case 3: The 25-Year-Old with Discharge

Scenario: *A 25-year-old woman presents with a complaint of abnormal vaginal discharge that is foul-smelling and associated with discomfort during urination.*

She also reports some pelvic discomfort and recent unprotected sexual activity.

- **Red Flags**:
  - Malodorous vaginal discharge
  - Associated pelvic discomfort or dyspareunia
  - Recent unprotected sexual activity
- **Differential Diagnosis**:
  - **Bacterial vaginosis (BV)** (most common cause of foul-smelling discharge)
  - Vaginal candidiasis (yeast infection)
  - Sexually transmitted infections (STIs), e.g., chlamydia or gonorrhoea
  - Trichomoniasis
- **Next Steps**:
  - Pelvic examination with speculum inspection for discharge type and visual inspection of the cervix
  - Wet mount microscopy of vaginal discharge to check for clue cells (for BV) or yeast (for candidiasis)
  - Nucleic acid amplification tests (NAATs) for STIs, particularly chlamydia and gonorrhoea
  - pH testing of vaginal discharge (pH >4.5 suggests BV or trichomoniasis)
- **Pearl**: **Bacterial vaginosis is often asymptomatic but may present with an unpleasant fishy odor. Treatment with metronidazole or clindamycin is effective.**
- **Pitfall**: Treating BV with antifungals due to misdiagnosis as a yeast infection, which can worsen symptoms.

- 4. Sudden Onset Of Severe Abdominal Pain With Nausea In The Mid-Cycle

Case 4: The 27-Year-Old with Acute Pain

Scenario: *A 27-year-old woman presents to the emergency department with sudden onset severe lower abdominal pain during the middle of her menstrual cycle.*

She also feels nauseous and has a mild fever. Her periods are regular, and she is not pregnant.

- **Red Flags**:
    - Sudden onset of severe abdominal pain (sharp, one-sided)
    - Mid-cycle timing (suggesting ovulation or other causes related to the menstrual cycle)
    - Nausea and fever
- **Differential Diagnosis**:
    - **Ovarian torsion** (most concerning due to risk of ischemia and loss of the ovary)
    - Ectopic pregnancy
    - Pelvic inflammatory disease (PID)
    - Ruptured ovarian cyst
- **Next Steps**:
    - Pelvic ultrasound to assess for ovarian cysts or signs of torsion
    - Serum beta-hCG to rule out ectopic pregnancy
    - Consider laparoscopy if ovarian torsion is suspected, as this is a surgical emergency
    - Administer pain relief and antiemetics if nausea is prominent

- **Pearl:** Ovarian torsion presents with sudden, severe pain and is a surgical emergency that requires early intervention to save the ovary.
- **Pitfall:** Delaying diagnosis and treatment of ovarian torsion, which may result in ovarian necrosis and loss.

- 5. Prolonged Menstrual Bleeding With Large Clots

Case 5: The 40-Year-Old with Heavy Periods

Scenario: *A 40-year-old woman presents with complaints of heavy menstrual bleeding lasting for more than 10 days.*

She passes large clots and has experienced fatigue and shortness of breath over the past few days.

She denies any abdominal pain or fever.

- **Red Flags:**
  - Prolonged and heavy menstrual bleeding (more than 7 days)
  - Passage of large clots and soaking through pads or tampons frequently
  - Symptoms of anemia (fatigue, shortness of breath)
- **Differential Diagnosis:**
  - **Uterine fibroids** (common cause of heavy menstrual bleeding)
  - Endometrial hyperplasia
  - Endometrial carcinoma
  - Coagulopathies (e.g., von Willebrand disease, platelet disorders)
- **Next Steps:**
  - Pelvic ultrasound to check for fibroids, adenomyosis, or other uterine pathology

- ◦ Endometrial biopsy if there are any concerns for malignancy or hyperplasia
- ◦ Lab tests to assess for anemia (CBC) and clotting disorders (e.g., platelet count, PT/INR)
- ◦ Hormonal management (e.g., progestins, IUD) or surgical options like myomectomy if fibroids are confirmed
- **Pearl: Heavy menstrual bleeding with clots often indicates uterine fibroids. However, malignancy should always be ruled out in women over 40 years old.**
- **Pitfall:** Failing to rule out endometrial carcinoma in women with abnormal bleeding, especially in those over 40, which can delay necessary interventions.

UROLOGY: RED FLAGS

- 1. Hematuria (Blood In Urine)

Case 1: The 60-Year-Old with Blood in Urine

Scenario: *A 60-year-old man presents with painless hematuria for the past 3 days.*

He noticed blood in his urine after using the toilet and is now worried, though he has no associated pain or other symptoms.

He has a history of smoking for 40 years but denies recent trauma or infections.

- **Red Flags**:
  - **Painless hematuria** in a patient over 50
  - History of **smoking** or occupational exposure (e.g., chemical exposure)
  - **No clear cause** of hematuria (not related to trauma, infections, or menstruation in females)
- **Differential Diagnosis**:
  - **Bladder cancer** (most concerning cause of painless hematuria in older adults)
  - Renal cell carcinoma
  - Urinary tract infections (UTIs) (usually painful, but can occasionally cause painless hematuria)
  - Nephrolithiasis (though usually associated with pain)
  - Benign prostatic hyperplasia (BPH) (in men)

- **Next Steps**:
  - **Urine dipstick** and **microscopic examination** for red blood cells
  - **Urinary cytology** to evaluate for malignant cells
  - **CT urography** or **Ultrasound** of the kidneys, bladder, and ureters
  - **Cystoscopy** (direct visualization of the bladder) if the imaging suggests bladder pathology or if hematuria persists
- **Pearl: Painless hematuria in patients over 50, especially with risk factors like smoking, is a strong indicator for bladder cancer until proven otherwise.**
- **Pitfall**: Assuming hematuria is benign (e.g., from a UTI or trauma) without proper investigation, especially in older patients with risk factors for cancer.

- 2. Acute Scrotal Pain

Case 2: The 25-Year-Old with Sudden Scrotal Pain

Scenario: *A 25-year-old male presents to the emergency department with sudden-onset severe scrotal pain on the left side.*

He denies any trauma but reports that the pain began suddenly while he was sitting down. He also feels nauseous and lightheaded.

On examination, the left testicle is very tender and slightly elevated.

- **Red Flags**:
    - **Sudden onset of severe scrotal pain**
    - **Nausea** and **vomiting** accompanying the pain
    - **Tender, swollen testicle** that is elevated
    - **Absence of cremasteric reflex** (if present, suggests testicular torsion)
- **Differential Diagnosis**:
    - **Testicular torsion** (most concerning, as it requires immediate intervention)
    - Epididymitis
    - Orchitis
    - Torsion of a testicular appendage (less severe than torsion but requires surgical evaluation)
- **Next Steps**:
    - **Urgent scrotal ultrasound** with Doppler to assess blood flow to the testicle
    - If torsion is confirmed, immediate **surgical detorsion** to preserve testicular viability
    - Administer **pain control** and **antiemetics** for nausea
- **Pearl: Testicular torsion is a surgical emergency**

—early intervention within 6 hours significantly increases the chances of saving the testicle.

- **Pitfall**: Delaying surgery or misdiagnosing testicular torsion as epididymitis or orchitis, which could lead to irreversible testicular damage.

- 3. Urinary Retention With Abdominal Distension

Case 3: The 70-Year-Old Male with Inability to Urinate

Scenario: *A 70-year-old man with a history of benign prostatic hyperplasia (BPH) presents with an inability to pass urine and significant lower abdominal distension.*

He is unable to void despite feeling the urge to urinate.

He reports occasional nocturia but has not experienced anything like this before.

- **Red Flags**:
  - **Inability to urinate** (acute urinary retention)
  - **Lower abdominal distension**
  - History of **benign prostatic hyperplasia (BPH)**
  - Recent **medication changes** or initiation of new drugs (e.g., antihistamines, decongestants)
- **Differential Diagnosis**:
  - **Benign prostatic hyperplasia (BPH)** causing obstruction
  - **Urinary tract infection (UTI)** with obstruction
  - Bladder stones or tumors
  - **Neurological causes** (e.g., spinal cord injury, multiple sclerosis, diabetic neuropathy)

- **Next Steps**:
  - ◦ **Bladder scan** or **urinary catheterization** to relieve the retention and assess post-void residual volume
  - ◦ **Digital rectal examination (DRE)** to assess for prostate enlargement
  - ◦ **Urinalysis** to check for signs of infection
  - ◦ **Urodynamic studies** if a neurological cause is suspected or if BPH treatment is ineffective
- **Pearl: Acute urinary retention can be life-threatening and needs prompt relief through catheterization. BPH is the most common cause in older men, but other causes must also be ruled out.**
- **Pitfall**: Failing to address the underlying cause of retention, especially in patients with BPH, and neglecting to consider other possible causes like infections or malignancy.

- 4. Painful Urination With Fever And Flank Pain

Case 4: The 40-Year-Old with Dysuria

Scenario: *A 40-year-old woman presents with a 2-day history of painful urination, fever, and sharp pain in her left flank.*

She also complains of chills and cloudy, foul-smelling urine. She has a history of recurrent UTIs.

- **Red Flags**:
  - ◦ **Fever** and **flank pain** in addition to dysuria
  - ◦ **Recent UTI history** or recurrent infections
  - ◦ **Chills and malaise** (indicating systemic infection)
- **Differential Diagnosis**:

- ◦ **Pyelonephritis** (upper urinary tract infection, most concerning due to potential renal damage)
- ◦ Cystitis (bladder infection)
- ◦ Kidney stones with secondary infection
- ◦ Renal abscess

- **Next Steps**:
  - ◦ **Urine culture** to identify the causative organism
  - ◦ **Blood cultures** if septicemia is suspected
  - ◦ **Renal ultrasound** or **CT scan** to assess for abscess or stones
  - ◦ Start **broad-spectrum IV antibiotics** while awaiting culture results, especially if sepsis is suspected

- **Pearl: Pyelonephritis can lead to sepsis and renal failure if not treated promptly with IV antibiotics and close monitoring.**
- **Pitfall**: Overlooking pyelonephritis as just a lower UTI and failing to escalate care to prevent sepsis.

- 5. Incontinence With Palpable Bladder

Case 5: The 45-Year-Old with Incontinence

Scenario: *A 45-year-old woman presents with complaints of urinary incontinence.*

She reports leakage of urine when she coughs, sneezes, or laughs.

On examination, her bladder is palpable above the symphysis pubis.

- **Red Flags**:
  - ◦ **Palpable bladder** (indicating bladder distension)

- New onset **incontinence** without any previous history
- **Sudden onset** of urinary symptoms, particularly in older women

- **Differential Diagnosis**:
  - **Overflow incontinence** (bladder overdistension leading to leakage)
  - Urge incontinence (overactive bladder)
  - Stress incontinence (often associated with pelvic floor weakness)
  - Neurological causes (e.g., spinal cord pathology, multiple sclerosis)

- **Next Steps**:
  - **Bladder scan** to confirm bladder distension and post-void residual volume
  - **Urodynamic studies** to assess bladder function and capacity
  - Referral to **urology** for further evaluation and management of overflow incontinence
  - Consider pelvic floor exercises or surgical intervention for pelvic organ prolapse or stress incontinence if indicated

- **Pearl: Overflow incontinence with a palpable bladder may indicate a neurological or obstructive cause and requires prompt urological evaluation.**

- **Pitfall**: Assuming all incontinence is due to pelvic floor weakness or stress incontinence without further evaluation for other causes like neurological or obstructive conditions.

INFECTIOUS DISEASES: RED FLAGS

- 1. Fever Of Unknown Origin (Fuo)

Case 1: The 35-Year-Old with Persistent Fever

Scenario: *A 35-year-old woman presents with a 2-week history of fever, chills, night sweats, and fatigue.*

She has no significant past medical history, and her physical exam is mostly unremarkable except for mild tachycardia.

She reports no recent travel, exposures, or known infections.

- **Red Flags**:
    - **Prolonged fever** (lasting > 3 weeks) without a clear source
    - **Systemic symptoms** like night sweats and fatigue
    - **Unexplained weight loss** or new-onset weakness
    - **No clear history** of infection or exposure
- **Differential Diagnosis**:
    - **Infectious causes** (e.g., tuberculosis, endocarditis, HIV/AIDS, abscesses)
    - **Non-infectious causes** (e.g., malignancies, autoimmune diseases like lupus, sarcoidosis, drug fevers)
    - **Tropical infections** (if recent travel is a factor)
    - **Viral infections** (e.g., Epstein-Barr virus, cytomegalovirus)

- **Next Steps**:
  - **Comprehensive work-up** including blood cultures, chest X-ray, and tuberculosis testing
  - **Autoimmune panel** if systemic signs (rash, joint pain) are present
  - **CT or MRI** of the abdomen and chest if signs of abscess or malignancy are suspected
  - **HIV testing** and specialized infectious disease screenings (e.g., tropical infections if relevant)
- **Pearl: Fever of unknown origin requires a systematic approach, with a thorough history and detailed physical exam. Rule out common infectious causes first, and be mindful of conditions like endocarditis and tuberculosis.**
- **Pitfall**: Rushing into empiric treatment without sufficient diagnostic workup can lead to misdiagnosis and delay appropriate therapy.

- 2. Sepsis (Severe Infection With Organ Dysfunction)

Case 2: The 60-Year-Old with Sepsis

Scenario: *A 60-year-old man with a history of diabetes mellitus presents with 2 days of fever, chills, and worsening confusion.*

On examination, he is febrile (39°C), tachycardic, and hypotensive (BP 85/50 mmHg).

He is lethargic and has decreased urine output.

A wound infection on his foot was noticed a few days ago.

- **Red Flags**:
  - **Fever, tachycardia, hypotension**
  - **Altered mental status** (confusion or delirium)
  - **Signs of organ dysfunction** (e.g., reduced urine output, liver enzyme abnormalities)
  - **Recent infection** (e.g., wound, urinary tract, lung)
- **Differential Diagnosis**:
  - **Sepsis** from a variety of sources (e.g., urinary tract infection, pneumonia, infected wound)
  - **Septic shock** (severe sepsis with hypotension despite fluids)
  - **Toxic shock syndrome** (especially with staphylococcal or streptococcal infections)
  - **Meningitis/encephalitis** (if neurological signs are prominent)
- **Next Steps**:
  - **Immediate IV fluids** (to address hypotension and support circulation)

- **Blood cultures** and **cultures from the suspected source** (e.g., wound, urine, sputum)
- **Broad-spectrum antibiotics** to cover likely pathogens (e.g., MRSA, gram-negative organisms)
- **Monitor vital signs** and consider **ICU admission** for intensive monitoring
- **Lactate levels** to assess severity and guide fluid resuscitation

- **Pearl: Sepsis is a medical emergency, and early recognition and rapid intervention with fluids, antibiotics, and source control can save lives.**
- **Pitfall**: Failing to initiate broad-spectrum antibiotics early in septic patients, especially if cultures are negative or pending.

- 3. Meningitis (Infection Of The Meninges)

Case 3: The 25-Year-Old with Headache and Stiff Neck

Scenario: *A 25-year-old male presents with a 3-day history of severe headache, fever, and nausea.*

He reports neck stiffness, photophobia, and confusion. On examination, he is febrile (38.5°C), and his neck is stiff.

He is also noted to have a petechial rash on his lower extremities.

- **Red Flags**:
  - **Fever, headache, neck stiffness**
  - **Photophobia** and **confusion** (signs of meningeal irritation)
  - **Petechial rash** (suggesting meningococcal infection)
  - **Altered mental status**
- **Differential Diagnosis**:
  - **Bacterial meningitis** (especially Neisseria meningitidis or Streptococcus pneumoniae)
  - **Viral meningitis** (e.g., enterovirus, herpes simplex virus)
  - **Tuberculous meningitis**
  - **Fungal meningitis** (e.g., Cryptococcus in immunocompromised patients)
- **Next Steps**:
  - **Lumbar puncture** for cerebrospinal fluid (CSF) analysis (cell count, glucose, protein, Gram stain, culture)
  - **Blood cultures** and **CT/MRI of the brain** before lumbar puncture if there is concern for increased intracranial pressure

- ○ **Empiric antibiotics** (e.g., ceftriaxone + vancomycin) and **antiviral** therapy (e.g., acyclovir for herpes simplex) if viral meningitis is suspected
- ○ **Isolation precautions** for meningococcal meningitis
- **Pearl: Bacterial meningitis is a medical emergency —early empiric antibiotics and supportive care are essential, especially in the case of meningococcal infection with its risk for rapid deterioration.**
- **Pitfall:** Delaying lumbar puncture or treatment due to concerns about increased intracranial pressure in suspected meningitis can lead to worsened outcomes.

- 4. Tuberculosis (Tb)

Case 4: The 40-Year-Old with Cough and Weight Loss

Scenario: *A 40-year-old man with a history of recent travel to India presents with a persistent cough, night sweats, and significant weight loss over the past 2 months.*

He denies hemoptysis but reports a low-grade fever and fatigue.

On examination, he is cachectic and has lymphadenopathy in the cervical region.

- **Red Flags**:
  - **Cough for > 3 weeks**
  - **Night sweats, weight loss, fever** (systemic symptoms)
  - **Travel history** to endemic areas (e.g., South Asia, Sub-Saharan Africa)
  - **Lymphadenopathy** and possible respiratory signs (e.g., crackles on chest auscultation)
- **Differential Diagnosis**:
  - **Pulmonary tuberculosis** (most likely in this case)
  - **Bronchitis or pneumonia** (though unlikely with this prolonged history)
  - **Lymphoma** (especially with constitutional symptoms)
  - **HIV-related opportunistic infections** (e.g., Pneumocystis pneumonia)
- **Next Steps**:
  - **Chest X-ray** to evaluate for lung lesions or cavitary changes consistent with TB
  - **Sputum smear** for acid-fast bacilli (AFB) and

culture for Mycobacterium tuberculosis

- Tuberculin skin test (TST) or interferon-gamma release assay (IGRA) for latent TB if active TB is ruled out

- Start antitubercular therapy (e.g., Rifampin, Isoniazid, Pyrazinamide, Ethambutol) if TB is confirmed

- Pearl: TB must be considered in any patient with a prolonged cough, weight loss, and systemic symptoms, especially if they have a history of travel to endemic areas.

- Pitfall: Missing the diagnosis of TB in patients without typical chest findings or not considering it in immunocompromised individuals.

- 5. Hiv/Aids

Case 5: The 30-Year-Old with Unexplained Weight Loss and Diarrhea

Scenario: *A 30-year-old male with a history of unprotected sexual intercourse presents with a 4-month history of weight loss, diarrhea, and night sweats.*

He has also noticed swollen lymph nodes in his neck.

He reports no known history of HIV, but has had multiple partners in the past year.

- **Red Flags**:
  - **Unexplained weight loss, diarrhea, night sweats**
  - **Lymphadenopathy** and other systemic symptoms
  - **Risk factors for HIV** (e.g., unprotected sexual contact, multiple partners)
- **Differential Diagnosis**:
  - **Acute HIV infection** (could present with "acute retroviral syndrome")
  - **AIDS-related opportunistic infections** (e.g., Cryptosporidiosis, Mycobacterium avium complex)
  - **Lymphoma** (especially in HIV-positive individuals)
  - **Tuberculosis** or **other infections**
- **Next Steps**:
  - **HIV testing** (rapid antigen/antibody test or HIV RNA PCR)
  - **CD4 count** and **viral load** to assess disease

stage

- ◦ **Screen for opportunistic infections** (e.g., stool cultures for parasites, chest X-ray for TB)
- ◦ **Start antiretroviral therapy (ART)** if HIV is confirmed
- **Pearl: Early HIV diagnosis allows for prompt treatment initiation, improving prognosis and preventing opportunistic infections.**
- **Pitfall**: Failing to test for HIV in high-risk patients, even in the absence of overt risk factors or symptoms.

ABOUT THE AUTHOR

Dr Essam Abdelhakim

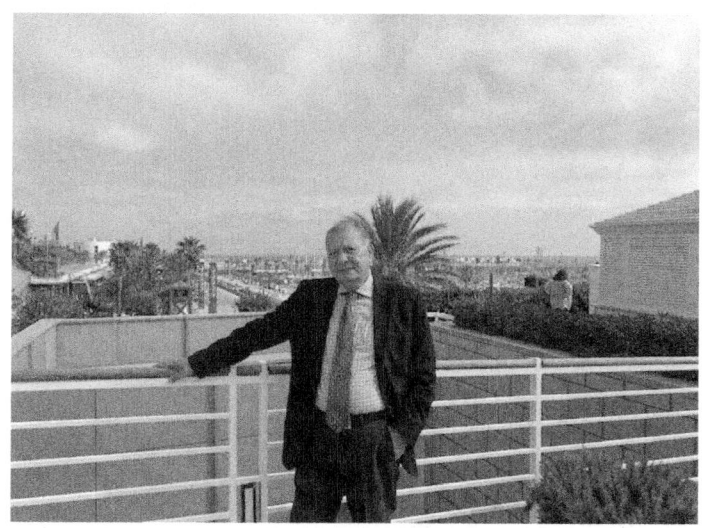

Senior Consultant and Expert in Medical Education

DISCLOSURE

Disclosure

This book has been created with the assistance of *Artificial Intelligence (AI) tools* and thoroughly reviewed and edited by the author to ensure clarity, relevance, and educational value.

While every effort has been made to provide accurate and up-to-date information, this content is intended solely for educational and informational purposes.

The author is a medical professional; however, the information provided in this book *is not a substitute for professional medical advice, diagnosis, or treatment.*

Readers are strongly advised to consult licensed healthcare providers or specialists for any medical concerns or conditions.

By using this book, **you acknowledge and agree** that the author shall not be held responsible or liable for any loss, damage, or harm whether physical, emotional, financial, or otherwise that may occur *as a result of the use or misuse of the information presented herein.*

Printed in Dunstable, United Kingdom

78749133R00087